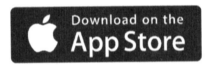
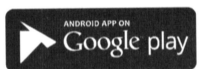

ISBN 978-1-332-31939-8
PIBN 10313446

1 MONTH OF
FREE
READING

at

www.ForgottenBooks.com

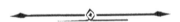

By purchasing this book you are eligible for one month membership to ForgottenBooks.com, giving you unlimited access to our entire collection of over 700,000 titles via our web site and mobile apps.

To claim your free month visit:

www.forgottenbooks.com/free313446

English
Français
Deutsche
Italiano
Español
Português

www.forgottenbooks.com

Mythology Photography **Fiction**
Fishing Christianity **Art** Cooking
Essays Buddhism Freemasonry
Medicine **Biology** Music **Ancient**
Egypt Evolution Carpentry Physics
Dance Geology **Mathematics** Fitness
Shakespeare **Folklore** Yoga Marketing
Confidence Immortality Biographies
Poetry **Psychology** Witchcraft
Electronics Chemistry History **Law**
Accounting **Philosophy** Anthropology
Alchemy Drama Quantum Mechanics
Atheism Sexual Health **Ancient History**
Entrepreneurship Languages Sport
Paleontology Needlework Islam
Metaphysics Investment Archaeology
Parenting Statistics Criminology
Motivational

BY THE SAME AUTHOR.

MANUAL OF DISEASES OF THE SKIN.   With an Analysis of Eight Thousand Consecutive Cases and a Formulary. $1.25.

NEUMANN'S HAND-BOOK OF SKIN DISEASES.   Translated, with Notes. Pp. 467. $4.00.

ARCHIVES OF DERMATOLOGY.   A Quarterly Journal of Skin and Venereal Diseases.   Vols. I. to VIII.   Vols. I. to IV., $3 00 per year ; Vols. V. to VIII., $4.00 per year.

THE SKIN IN HEALTH AND DISEASE.   Health Primer.   Pp. 145. Fifty Cents.

THE USE AND VALUE OF ARSENIC IN THE TREATMENT OF DISEASES OF THE SKIN.   Fifty Cents.   ·

IN PREPARATION :

PRINCIPLES AND PRACTICE OF DERMATOLOGY.   A Theoretical and Practical Treatise on Diseases of the Skin.   8vo.

ECZEMA

ND ITS MANAGEMENT

TICAL TREATISE BASED ON THE STUDY
OF THREE THOUSAND CASES OF
THE DISEASE

BY

DUNCAN BULKLEY, A.M., M.D.,

THE NEW YORK SKIN AND CANCER HOSPITAL; ATTENDING PHYSICIAN FOR SKIN AND
DISEASES AT THE NEW YORK HOSPITAL, OUT-PATIENT DEPARTMENT; DERMATOLOGIST
HOSPITAL FOR RUPTURED AND CRIPPLED; DERMATOLOGIST TO THE MANHATTAN
ND EAR HOSPITAL; LATE PHYSICIAN TO THE SKIN DEPARTMENT, DEMILT DIS-
PENSARY, NEW YORK; LATE EDITOR OF THE "ARCHIVES OF DERMATOLOGY;"
TRANSLATOR WITH NOTES OF "NEUMANN'S HAND-BOOK OF SKIN DIS-
EASES;" AUTHOR OF "THE SKIN IN HEALTH AND DISEASE,"
PERMANENT MEMBER OF THE AMERICAN MEDICAL ASSO-
CIATION; FELLOW OF THE AMERICAN ACADEMY OF
MEDICINE; FELLOW OF THE NEW YORK
ACADEMY OF MEDICINE, ETC.

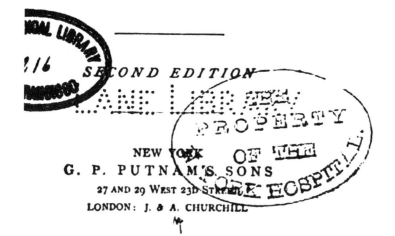

SECOND EDITION

NEW YORK
G. P. PUTNAM'S SONS
27 AND 29 WEST 23D STREET
LONDON: J. & A. CHURCHILL

LANE LIBRARY

Press of
G. P. Putnam's Sons
New York

TO THE

MEMORY OF MY FATHER

THE LATE

HENRY D. BULKLEY, M. D.,

FIRST PRESIDENT OF THE NEW YORK DERMATOLOGICAL SOCIETY,

LATE PRESIDENT OF THE NEW YORK ACADEMY OF MEDICINE,

AND ONE OF THE FIRST TO STUDY AND LECTURE

ON DERMATOLOGY IN THIS COUNTRY, THIS

VOLUME IS AFFECTIONATELY

DEDICATED.

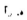

to make more clear the practical portions. As in the former edition, little attempt has been made to refer to particular opinions of other writers, for reasons stated in the preface to that edition.

In conclusion the author would solicit a careful study of the whole work, that the reader may understand the subject fully, for only thus can eczema be intelligently and successfully treated. With careful, thorough, and judicious management, there are few of the chronic diseases which yield such satisfactory and often brilliant results as eczema, whereas with routine and imperfect treatment it can resist cure in a manner unexcelled by few maladies.

4 EAST 37TH STREET, NEW YORK.

PREFACE.

THE aim of the following pages has been to present the general practitioner with as clear a guide as possible to the recognition and management of eczema. To this end the author has endeavored to give minute directions in reference to many of the features which daily experience has shown to be of great importance in regard to the disease, and to meet the difficulties which have presented themselves in practice and which have developed from contact with physicians in consultation and in class instruction. He has further endeavored to answer many questions which have been put to him from time to time, both by physicians and patients, and which have been jotted down during the past two years while this work was in progress.

The book, therefore, is a personal one, representing the views and experience of the writer; and omission of frequent and particular reference to the opinions and statements of other writers has not occurred from any neglect or from any disregard of them, but has resulted from a desire that the pages should not be occupied with references which might not be required by the practitioner. The author acknowledges fully the special writings of Wilson, Anderson, and Fox on Eczema, and also the assistance gained from text-books on Dermatology, especially from such classical works as those of Duhring in this country, and Hebra, Wilson, Fox, and Hardy abroad. But it is often difficult for one much occupied with a subject to state definitely where or how his knowledge has been gained, and in the present writing it would be impossible to define how far the influence of this or that writer had modified or altered the views here put forth.

In regard to the emphasis which is laid upon the constitutional origin and relations of eczema, it is proper to state that, although the writer was educated in the Vienna School, and although local pathology was further inculcated by his own translation of Neumann's Handbook of Skin Diseases, he has still felt constrained to urge to the utmost the constitutional, as opposed to purely local pathology and treatment, because he is confident that success in dealing with the disease can be thus best attained. The teachings of the late Dr. H. D. Bulkley, together with hospital and dispensary practice in general diseases, coupled with close observation and study of skin diseases in private and public practice, have led the writer to take the constitutional view of eczema and many other diseases of the skin, which view further experience and study daily confirms.

In the complete consideration of the subject in hand it was necessary to have a certain amount of repetition, for which indulgence is craved. The different chapters of this book have been written at intervals during the past several years, and many of them have been presented before different medical bodies as separate essays, and the writer has been able to profit by the ensuing discussions. Chapter VI, upon the Constitutional or Local nature of eczema is largely a reprint of the essay which the author was invited to read before the International Medical Congress at Philadelphia in 1876, to open the discussion upon the question, "Are Eczema and Psoriasis local diseases of the skin, or are they manifestations of a constitutional disorder?" Many of the sections have already appeared in print in the Medical Journals, but they have been worked over and the whole put into a shape which will, it is hoped, make it valuable both as a work for study and also for reference in time of need. There will, therefore, be found some repetition in the different chapters, in reference to the matters of etiology, diagnosis, and treatment; but this has appeared to be unavoidable, as it was desired that each chapter on regional eczema should be as complete as possible.

In regard to the Chapter on Therapeutics, giving formulæ, a word may be said. While it is acknowledged that it is better to have principles upon which practice can be based, yet in the treatment of diseases of the skin, and especially of eczema, there is so much uncertainty in the minds of those who have not had much experience in this direction that it was thought best to give the exact formulæ which had been found of value in practice, hoping that if they were not employed they might still convey a hint which might help in selecting and applying a remedy for the diseased skin.

The basis of this volume is an essay on "The Management of Eczema" which the author read before the American Medical Association in 1874. A small edition was reprinted and put on sale ; this was exhausted very shortly and there have been so many demands for it that a more full and complete treatise on the same subject has seemed to be demanded. While not claiming to be exhaustive, the author believes that he has in the following pages given the facts in regard to eczema so fully that a careful study of them will enable most physicians to manage with success this disease, which is very frequent and yet which does not seem to be thoroughly understood by every practitioner.

4 East 37th Street, New York.

CONTENTS.

CHAPTER IX.

CHAPTER X.

CHAPTER XI.

CHAPTER XII.

CHAPTER XIII.

CHAPTER XIV.

CHAPTER XV.

CHAPTER XVI.

ECZEMA AND ITS MANAGEMENT.

CHAPTER I.

GENERAL CONSIDERATIONS.—DEFINITION OF ECZEMA.—NOS-
OLOGY OF ECZEMA.

ECZEMA has been rightly called the keystone of Dermatology, and he who masters its management is not only
skilled in regard to treating the most common and distressing of all cutaneous diseases, but has acquired a
knowledge of the principles of dermatological practice
which will assist in the treatment of very many, if not all,
other maladies of the skin.

Assuming a multitude of forms, and appearing under
the most varied circumstances, difficulties continually arise
as to the diagnosis of individual cases, while exactly the
proper management of a single severe or obstinate attack
of eczema may at times give the physician more perplexity
than a score of general cases. A careful study of the disease is, therefore, a subject of vital interest to every practitioner, for eczema attacks all classes and conditions of
persons, from the cradle to the grave, and is an affection
about which advice is continually asked. Judging, however, from the numbers of cases of eczema which exist on
all sides, many of them of great duration, it would appear
to be a malady which is not, in the main, well understood, and moreover, one which often does not receive the

careful consideration and thought which it merits from the distress it occasions.

Undoubtedly many patients are themselves to blame in part, for the severity and persistency of their complaint. Eczema frequently being a chronic state, they too often become weary, and chafe under the restraints and annoyances of treatment long before the disease is cured, and relapse follows relapse, relief being sought for only when there is distress from the itching or pain, or when the eruption becomes troublesome upon exposed parts. But on the other hand many cases are also too lightly regarded by the physician, and are thus suffered to run on for weeks, months, or even years, with little or no treatment other than palliative measures, no attempt being made to alter the conditions of life upon which the disease depends.

Oft times the opinion is expressed that the eruption will cease of itself when certain periods of life are past, as nursing, dentition, puberty, the menopause, etc., and so the case is neglected until the eczematous habit is acquired to such a degree as to render the disease very much more obstinate. Many cases, again, are left untreated from the fear that if the eruption is cured in one part it will go to another, or from a dread lest the disease may "strike in," or be "driven in," and the eruption is often considered salutary, and is thought to be serviceable in relieving the system of some supposed peccant material. It would hardly seem necessary to mention such points in the present enlightened age, were it not that they are constantly brought to my notice by physicians as well as patients; they are alluded to solely to deny the foundation upon which any such fears may rest, as will abundantly appear elsewhere.

The hold which this idea, namely, that a disease on the skin is the outward manifestation of some poison seeking exit, had upon a past, unenlightened, medical opinion, is shown in the very name given to the disease under consideration, to wit, *eczema*, from the Greek ἐκζειν, to boil over. The same thought is also expressed in the general term "eruption," from the Latin *erumpere*, to burst forth.

Eczema, as will be seen, is an exceedingly common affection, and forms a large share of the cases of skin disease ordinarily met with in general practice. It is found in all countries with almost the same frequency, and occurs under the most varying circumstances, exhibiting widely different appearances in different cases.

While, however, eczema is a most protean disease, presenting at times almost all the lesions which the skin is capable of, it will yet be seen that the term is not loosely applied, but represents a well-defined affection of the skin, with many constitutional relations, which are quite as important to recognize as the lesions themselves. Notwithstanding this fact, much confusion still exists in the minds of many in regard to this disease, and many eruptions are called eczema in a comprehensive way; often, indeed, the term is used simply as a synonym for cutaneous disease in general, without any attempt to discriminate between the lesions proper to it, and to other diseases of the skin.

Many cases also of simple dermatitis, transient in character, due wholly to local causes, are also often wrongly classed as eczema; as, for instance, the eruptions produced on the scalp by pediculi, or on the face or hands by poison ivy, etc.

In the older works the term eczema was used somewhat more vaguely that at present, and cases which were previously included under eczema are now well recognized as distinct affections, such as lichen planus, and dermatitis; on the other hand, many other cases which would formerly have been named chronic erythema or erysipelas, lichen, and impetigo, are now acknowledged to be eczema.

... strated that the les...
... that we are no longer ...
... element in every inst...
... lesions are secondar...
... disease state, whose ca...
... and capillary disturba...
... cess in the skin and its i...
... best understood by regar...
... inflammation of the skin. qu...
... as presented elsewhere in t...
... the permanent cure of eczema i...
... its constitutional nature, its in-
... difying elements, which will be

... be defined as *a non-contagious,*
... skin, of constitutional origin.
... manifesting any or all the
... one or in succession, and accom-
... ing.

... phenomena being nerve and capil-
... process may remain in the erythe-
... skin lesion be aborted, as far as re-
... case, and the threatened eruption
... further advance. Or the capillary
... a certain amount of fluid may
... organized, and the chronic erythe-
... sults. Or, there may occur so much
... cles are formed, and when these rupt-
... fluid exudes, which stiffens linen, and
... scales and crusts. If the inflammation
... papules are formed. In the more
... exuded fluid does not reach the surface,
... the meshes of the skin, and, becoming
... stitutes what is known as the infiltration or
... of eczema, which may then crack and give

Clinical research has demonstrated that the lesions of eczema are multiform, and that we are no longer to look for the vesicle as a necessary element in every instance of this eruption. The external lesions are secondary elements or results of a deeper disease state, whose earliest local manifestations are nerve and capillary disturbance.

The actual disease process in the skin and its immediate local treatment will be best understood by regarding eczema as a dermatitis, an inflammation of the skin, quite analogous to inflammation as presented elsewhere in the human system. But, for the permanent cure of eczema it is essential to remember its constitutional nature, its internal relations and its modifying elements, which will be considered later.

Eczema, therefore, may be defined as *a non-contagious, inflammatory disease of the skin, of constitutional origin, acute or chronic in character, manifesting any or all the results of inflammation at once or in succession, and accompanied by burning and itching.*

The earliest local phenomena being nerve and capillary disturbance, the process may remain in the erythematous stage, and the skin lesion be aborted, as far as relates to its active increase, and the threatened eruption may subside without further advance. Or the capillary dilatation may continue, a certain amount of fluid may transude and become organized, and the chronic erythematous eczema results. Or, there may occur so much exudation that vesicles are formed, and when these rupture a peculiar glairy fluid exudes, which stiffens linen, and tends to dry into scales and crusts. If the inflammation is less active only papules are formed. In the more chronic cases the exuded fluid does not reach the surface, but is retained in the meshes of the skin, and, becoming organized, constitutes what is known as the infiltration or thickening of eczema, which may then crack and give great distress. The special features belonging to different phases of the eruption will be subsequently described.

While eczema was defined as an inflammation of the skin, it differs from all other dermal inflammations, as erythema, erysipelas, acne, psoriasis, etc., in its exudative feature, in which it stands alone and resembles the catarrhal affections of the mucous membranes. This catarrhal exudation, previously alluded to as stiffening linen, has led certain writers to call eczema a catarrhal disease of the skin, a clinical point rightly taken and one which it is well to constantly bear in mind. The stages of heat and dryness, subsequent tumefaction, and later free discharge, occurring in an ordinary mucous catarrh, all find their counterpart in acute eczema, while the thickening of the membrane and the constant exudation and irritation of chronic mucous inflammation answer to certain chronic eczematous states.

It is also to be remembered that although eczema differs from ordinary inflammation of the skin, or dermatitis excited by local irritants, it is often very difficult to distinguish between the two early in the attack. Pediculi upon the scalp give rise to an irritation which induces scratching, and an artificial eruption is then set up, composed of pustules and raw points covered with crusts, which often closely resembles a pustular eczema of the scalp. But the former eruption is not eczema, it is simply a dermatitis depending wholly on the local cause of the pediculi, and disappearing entirely when they are removed. The same is true in regard to eruptions caused by body lice, and pediculi pubis, also of the eruptions seen in scabies. Other agencies may likewise cause inflammation of the skin which may closely resemble that of eczema ; such are heat and cold, animal poisons, also such vegetable matters as croton oil, savin, poison ivy, and arnica, together with mineral substances as tartar emetic, aniline dyes, etc.

Although these eruptions are not eczema, they may become the starting point of true eczema, which may then remain, and relapse again and again without recognizable local cause.

Eczema, then, is not purely a local disease of the skin, but is a state or condition of the system of which the skin lesions are the outward manifestations, as joint inflammation is one of the indications of the gouty state. The real nature of the systemic changes which underlie the skin disorder will be discussed later, and will be found to be essentially one of debility; in many cases the gouty habit appears to be at the bottom of it, in others a scrofulous or strumous condition, in still other instances the whole difficulty can be apparently traced to nerve disorder or depression.

In regard to the nosological position of eczema, it is classed according to the appearances of the eruption and not at all with reference to its nature or causes. Comparatively few diseases of the skin have as yet been grouped etiologically, and the dermatological world has largely accepted a classification based mainly upon pathological states, with a few groups of diseases made upon other grounds. The details of classification cannot be entered into here, but the following scheme, simplified from that of Hebra, represents in the main the principles which are widely accepted, and serves to locate eczema among the many eruptions to which the skin is subject.

The inflammatory element has been emphasized and also the polymorphous character of its lesions, and these features form the basis on which its nosological position is decided. It belongs, therefore, in the annexed scheme of classification, in the fourth class, among exudative or inflammatory affections. Here it is found, fourteenth in order, in the second division, namely, among diseases of internal or of local origin ; and here again it forms a sixth group, with dermatitis, which so often resembles it in the multiform a earances which both ma resent.

CLASSIFICATION OF DISEASES OF THE SKIN.

CLASS   I.   Morbi cutis parasitici.   Parasitic Affections.
"   II.   Morbi glandularum cutis.   Glandular Affections.
"   III.   Neuroses.   Neurotic Affections.
"   IV.   Exsudationes.   Exudative or Inflammatory Affections.
"   V.   Hæmorrhagiæ.   Hæmorrhagic Affections.
"   VI.   Hypertrophiæ.   Hypertrophic Affections.
"   VII.   Atrophiæ.   Atrophic Affections.
"   VIII.   Neoplasmata.   New Formations.

Class I. Morbi cutis parasitici. Parasitic Affections.

A. VEGETA- BLE.

1. Tinea trichophytina (or trichophytosis) (parasite—Trichophyton tonsurans).
   - corporis (or tinea circinata).
   - capitis (or tinea tonsurans).
   - barbæ (or sycosis parasitica).
   - cruris (or eczema marginatum).

2. Tinea favosa (or favus) (parasite—Achorion Schœnleinii).

3. Tinea versicolor (or pityriasis versicolor) (parasite—Microsporon furfur).

B. ANIMAL.

1. Phthiriasis (or pediculosis)
   - corporis
   - capitis
   - pubis
   (parasite—Pediculus).

2. Scabies (parasite—Acarus scabiei).

Class II. Morbi glandularum cutis. Glandular Affections.

A. DISEASES OF THE SEBACEOUS GLANDS.

I. Due to faulty secretion or excretion of sebaceous matter.

1. Acne sebacea
   - oleosa
   - cerea
   - cornea
   (or seborrhœa).

2. Acne punctata
   - nigra (or comedo).
   - albida (or milium).

3. Acne molluscum (or molluscum sebaceum).

II. Due to inflammation of sebaceous glands with surrounding tissue.

4. Acne simplex (or vulgaris).
5. Acne indurata.
6. Acne rosacea.

B. DISEASES OF THE SWEAT- GLANDS.

I. As to quantity of secretion.
1. Hyperidrosis.
2. Anidrosis.

II. As to quality of secretion.
3. Bromidrosis.
4. Chromidrosis.

III. With retention of secretion.
5. Dysidrosis.
6. Sudamina.

Class III. Neuroses. Neurotic Affections.

1. Zoster (herpes zoster or zona).
2. Pruritus.
3. Dermatalgia.
4. Hyperæsthesia cutis.
5. Anæsthesia cutis.
6. Dystrophia cutis (or trophic disturbances).

Class IV. Exsudationes. Exudative or Inflammatory Affections.

A. Induced by Infection or Contagion.

1. Rubeola (or measles).
2. Röthełn (or German measles).
3. Scarlatina.
4. Variola.
5. Varicella.
6. Vaccinia.
7. Syphilis.
8. Pustula maligna.
9. Equinia (or glanders).
10. Diphtheritis cutis.
11. Erysipelas.

B. Of Internal or Local Origin.

I. Erythematous.
1. Roseola.
2. Erythema — simplex. multiforme. nodosum.
3. Urticaria.

II. Papular.
4. Lichen — simplex. planus. ruber. scrofulosus.
5. Prurigo.

III. Vesicular.
6. Herpes — febrilis. iris. progenitalis. gestationis.

IV. Bullous.
7. Hydroa.
8. Pemphigus — vulgaris. foliaceus.
9. Pompholyx (or cheiro-pompholyx).

V. Pustular.
10. Sycosis (or folliculitis pilorum).
11. Impetigo.
12. Impetigo contagiosa.
13. Ecthyma.

VI. Multiform, i. e., erythematous, papular, vesicular, pustular, etc.
14. Eczema.
15. Dermatitis — calorica. venenata. traumatica. medicamentosa.

VII. Squamous.
16. Dermatitis exfoliativa (or pityriasis rubra)..
17. Psoriasis.
18. Pityriasis capitis.

VIII. Phlegmonous.
19. Furunculus (furunculosis).
20. Anthrax.
21. Abscessus.
22. Hordeolum.

IX. Ulcerative.
23. Onychia.
24. Ulcus — simplex. venereum.

Class V. Hæmorrhagiæ. Hæmorrhagic Affections.

1. Purpura { simplex. / papulosa. / rheumatica (or peliosis rheumatica). / hæmorrhagica.

2. Hæmatidrosis (or bloody sweat).
3. Scorbutus.

Class VI. Hypertrophiæ. Hypertrophic Affections.

A. OF PIGMENT. { 1. Lentigo. / 2. Chloasma. / 3. Melanoderma.
4. Nævus pigmentosus.
5. Morbus Addisonii.

B. OF EPIDERMIS AND PAPILLÆ. { 1. Keratosis pilaris (or lichen pilaris). / 2. Ichthyosis. / 3. Cornu cutaneum. / 4. Clavus. / 5. Tylosis (or callositas).
6. Verruca { vulgaris. / senilis. / acuminata. / necrogenica.

C. OF CONNECTIVE TISSUE. { 1. Scleroderma. / 2. Morphœa. / 3. Sclerema neonatorum.
4. Elephantiasis (Arabum).
5. Dermatolysis.
6. Frambœsia (or yaws).

D. OF HAIR. 1. Hirsuties. 2. Nævus pilosus.
E. OF NAIL. 1. Onychogryphosis. 2. Onychauxis.

Class VII. Atrophiæ. Atrophic Affections.

A. OF PIGMENT. { 1. Albinismus. / 2. Leucoderma (or vitiligo). / 3. Canities.

B. OF CORIUM. { 1. Atrophia cutis { propria. / linearis (or striæ atrophicæ). / maculosa (or maculæ atrophicæ). / 2. Atrophia senilis.

C. OF HAIR. { 1. Alopecia. 2. Alopecia areata. / 3. Trichorexis nodosa (or atrophia pilorum propria). / 4. Fragilitas crinium.

D. OF NAIL. Onychatrophia.

Class VIII. Neoplasmata. New Formations.

I. BENIGN NEW FORMATIONS.

A. OF CONNECTIVE TISSUE. { 1. Keloid. 2. Fibroma (or molluscum fibrosum). / 3. Xanthoma (xanthelasma or vitiligoidea).

B. OF FATTY TISSUE. Lipoma.

C. OF GRANULATION TISSUE. { 1. Lupus { vulgaris. / erythematosus. 2. Scrofuloderma. / 3. Rhinoscleroma.

D. OF BLOOD-VESSELS. { 1. Nævus vasculosus. / 2. Angioma (or telangiectasis).

E. OF LYMPHATICS. { 1. Lymphadenoma cutis. / 2. Lymphangioma cutis.

F. OF NERVES. Neuroma cutis.

II. MALIGNANT NEW FORMATIONS.

1. Lepra. { maculosa / tuberculosa / anæsthetica } (leprosy, or elephantiasis Græcorum).

2. Carcinoma.
3. Epithelioma (and rodent ulcer).
4. Sarcoma. { idiopathicum. / pigmentosum (or melanosis).

CHAPTER II.

THAT eczema is by far the most frequent of all skin diseases none will deny, but its relative frequency as compared with other skin affections is by no means decided. Statistics vary considerably on this point, some making the proportion of cases of eczema in miscellaneous skin cases very low, while others place the ratio as high as forty or fifty per cent of all cases of skin diseases applying for treatment, in special practice.

The relative numbers of patients applying for the relief of eczema must differ somewhat according to the source whence the statistics are drawn. Thus, the number will be found much greater in any statistics where young children are included, for by far the larger share of young children presenting diseases of the skin are found to have eczema; in many public institutions, all children under a certain age are sent to a special children's department, and thus the whole number of skin cases do not come under the observation of the one in charge of the dermatological department.

In Hebra's skin clinic in Vienna, no children under four or five years of age appear; hence the ratio of eczema to other diseases is very much smaller than in other places. Taking the recent reports of his clinic for two years, we have 517 cases of eczema among 3,217 of general skin disease, or only a trifle over 16 per cent.

Neumann gives a yet smaller proportion in former years, stating that among 29,535 patients with skin disease, attending Hebra's clinic, there were only 2,195 cases of eczema, or not quite *eight* per cent.

This, however, cannot be taken as a fair representation of the frequency of eczema in Germany, for, of 2,592 skin patients reported by Veiel, there were 717 cases of eczema, or a trifle over 27 per cent.

Among 9,809 cases of skin disease reported by Englested in Copenhagen, Denmark, there were 1,724 of eczema, or 17½ per cent. In Glasgow, McCall Anderson gives 6,446 cases of eczema in 21,859 dispensary cases, or almost 30 per cent, and 34.8 per cent for private cases. Wilson makes the percentage to be 33½ among the wealthier classes, in London.

In this country, among 52,214 cases of miscellaneous skin diseases, collected by the statistical committee of the American Dermatological Association, occurring in New York, Boston, Philadelphia, Baltimore, St. Louis, and Chicago, during the last few years, there were found 16,205 cases of eczema, or over thirty-one per cent.

My own statistics, gathered from personal cases observed in private practice, also at the Demilt Dispensary, and the out-patient departments of the New York and Bellevue Hospitals, give 3,000 cases of eczema in a total of 8,661 cases of miscellaneous skin diseases, or a percentage of 34.63. Of these, 1,200 cases of eczema were seen in private practice occurring among 3,419 general skin cases, and 1,800 cases in public practice, among 5,242 cases. The ratio of eczema to other skin diseases was almost the same in both classes of practice, namely, 35.09 per cent. of private cases, and 34.33 in public cases.

Eczema may, therefore, be safely regarded as forming at least one-third of all cases of skin diseases, as shown by statistics, although it is more than likely that the real proportion is still greater : probably nearly one half of all those afflicted with cutaneous diseases have eczema.

Eczema affects the sexes almost equally. Thus, of the 3,000 cases there were 1,583 males to 1,417 females ; in the statistics from private practice, males formed 59.9 per cent. of the 1,200 cases, while in public practice, the females were slightly in excess, presenting exactly 52 per cent. ; in the total number the males formed 52.76 per cent.

Hebra gives the proportion of male to female patients with eczema as two to one. This may possibly have to do with peculiarities of the disease in Vienna, though more probably the difference between his figures and mine may be accounted for by the peculiarities of his clinic ; in so public a place the females may be less disposed to appear than in the more private clinics of our dispensaries and hospitals, and in consultation practice.

The following table will exhibit the ages of the patients when first coming under observation :

TABLE I.—AGES OF 3,000 PATIENTS WITH ECZEMA.

AGES.	MALES.	FEMALES.	TOTAL.
6 months and under....................	69	53	122
6 " to 1 year	50	43	93
1 year to 2 years	94	68	162
2 years " 3 "	74	69	143
3 " " 4 "	47	48	95
4 " " 5 "	29	32	61
Total infantile eczema............	363	313	676
5 years to 10 years....................	105	126	231
10 " 20 "	105	188	293
20 " 30 "	210	206	416
30 " 40 "	250	166	416
40 " 50 "	214	188	402
50 " 60 "	196	137	333
60 " 70 "	103	68	171
70 " 80 "	34	18	52
80 " 90 "	3	4	7
90 " 100 "		1	1
Unknown age.........................		2	2
	1583	1417	3000

It is not possible from the data collected to make an accurate statement in regard to the ages at which eczema first appears ; a subsequent table will give the duration of the disease in those cases in private practice where this could be determined with sufficient exactness.

It will be seen from this that no age is spared, from the cradle to the grave, although certain periods are much more subject to the disease than others. The youngest patient recorded in private practice was a male infant four weeks old, although in public practice several still younger subjects were seen, some even as young as two weeks of age. The oldest private patient with eczema was a male aged 90; the oldest in public practice, a female over 90 years of age.

Almost one-quarter of the entire number of cases, namely 676, were under five years of age, coming within the definition of infantile eczema ; and of these it will be observed ,that 520, or more than three-quarters of all the cases, were less than three years old, indicating in a measure the influence of dentition in the production of the disease. Between three and four years of age the number diminishes, so that between the ages of four and five not one third of the number of cases are recorded which are found during the first years of life.

Taking the decades, 907 cases were observed in the first ten years of life and only 293 cases in the second decade, namely, from ten to twenty years of age. The proportion then increases in the next two decades very considerably, so that between 20 and 30, and 30 and 40 years of age we meet with the largest number, except during the first ten years of life ; and probably, considering the relative proportion of persons living at this period of life compared with the number during the first ten years, the disease is almost if not quite as frequent then as during infancy. Among my private cases, the decade between

30 and 40 furnished actually a larger number of cases than that from birth to ten years of age.

The annexed table shows the ages of the private cases divided into periods of five years each.

TABLE II.—AGES OF 1200 ECZEMA PATIENTS IN PRIVATE PRACTICE.

AGES.	MALES.	FEMALES.	TOTAL.
6 months and under......................	32	16	48
6 months to 1 year......................	20	8	28
1 year to 2 years	22	13	35
2 years " 3 "	15	16	31
3 " " 4 "	8	12	20
4 " " 5 "	1	7	8
Total infantile eczema...........	98	72	170
5 years to 10 years......................	21	20	41
10 " 15 "	13	25	38
15 " 20 "	21	45	66
20 " 25 "	34	48	82
25 " 30 "	56	53	109
30 " 35 "	78	34	112
35 " 40 "	75	34	109
40 " 45 "	76	32	108
45 " 50 "	60	36	96
50 " 55 "	47	25	72
55 " 60 "	58	19	77
60 " 65 "	30	19	49
65 " 70 "	27	8	35
70 " 75 "	18	6	24
75 " 80 "	6	3	9
80 " 85 "		2	2
85 " 90 "	1		1
	719	481	1200

In regard to the duration of the disease, a large number of the cases here analyzed had lasted many months or even years before coming under observation; comparatively few examples of really acute eruptions appear here. Undoubtedly, however, statistics collected from the practice of family physicians would show quite different figures, as they frequently see the case at the beginning of the eruption, while those in special consulting practice are very commonly called upon after the disease has lasted some time and has proved rebellious. By the duration of the disease is not meant the length of time which any one attack or exacerbation of the eruption has lasted, but the period during which the patient has suffered from the malady to a greater or less degree.

Records from public practice would be very unreliable in this regard, and the following table is taken from over a thousand private patients in the higher walks of life, in whom the matter was carefully investigated and recorded at the time of the first visit.

TABLE III.—DURATION OF ECZEMA IN 1055 PRIVATE CASES.

DURATION.	MALES.	FEMALES.	TOTAL.
Under 1 week	5	3	8
1 week	5	7	12
2 weeks..............................	17	12	29
3 "	16	10	26
1 month	16	14	30
2 months	51	25	76
3 "	31	25	56
4 "	25	18	43
5 "	12	6	18
6 "	28	22	50
6 " to 1 year.....................	66	57	123
1 year to 2 years	74	55	129
2 years to 3 years	50	38	88
3 " 4 "	25	23	48
4 " 5 "	25	9	34
5 " 10 "	50	29	79
10 " 15 "	31	21	52
15 " 20 "	18	7	25
Chronic.............................	89	40	129
	634	421	1055

It will be noticed that a number are recorded simply as " chronic." This indefinite term refers to possibly more or less years than those which were definitely stated of other patients. A number of cases have occurred where the disease had lasted since infancy, the patient being hardly, if ever, free from the eruption; in several instances the duration had been from infancy or childhood up to fifty or more years of age. One half the cases had lasted over six months before they came under observation.

The frequency with which the disease attacks various portions of the body may be of some interest, and is exhibited in the following table. The items of this will be more or less noticed when the varieties of eczema in its several localities are taken up separately.

TABLE IV.—LOCATION OF THE ERUPTION.

LOCATION.	MALE	FEMALE.	TOTAL.
Head	125	104	229
Face	179	171	350
Neck	17	34	51
Tongue	1		1
Upper extremities	71	52	123
Hands	104	88	192
Body	39	33	72
Thighs and Legs	141	51	192
Feet	29	13	42
Genitals	134	20	154
General	82	41	123
	922	607	1529 .

Much has been said in reference to the heredity of eczema, and both sides of the question have found warm advocates, and the impression is very general that the disease is very commonly acquired by transmission. The following table shows how small a proportion exhibited this element among seven hundred and sixty-five private patients in regard to whom this matter was investigated.

TABLE V.—RELATIVES OF 765 PRIVATE PATIENTS WITH ECZEMA.

	FREE.	AFFECTED.	TOTAL.
Parents	1304	226	1530
Children	849	100	949
Brothers and sisters	959	220	1179
Grandparents	4	43	47
Uncles and aunts	5	39	44
Cousins		13	13
Grandchildren	8	5	13
Nieces	1	2	3
	3130	648	3778

It will be seen here that out of 3,778 relatives of 765 private eczema patients but 648 were said to be affected—only about 17 per cent. Of 1,530 parents only 226 were said to have eczema; of over 900 children, but 100, or one-tenth; of 1,179 brothers and sisters, 220, or less than eighteen per cent.; a total of 546 among 3,658 near relatives, or one-sixth of all. The figures relating to the remaining relatives mentioned in the table have little bearing in this connection; for, as is observed, no negative statements which could be relied on were obtained as to those who were free from the disease.

I must state that I have very little belief in the heredity of eczema as a disease, although the habit or condition which predisposes thereto, namely, the gouty, strumous, and nervous states may be and undoubtedly are transmitted. I have sought for evidence of heredity among large numbers of patients in public practice, and in addition to the constant denial always obtained in regard to the existence of other cases in the family, I have constantly remarked to those about me how very rare it was to see a mother and child both affected, and how constantly it was observed that other members of the family accompanying eczema patients were entirely free from the disease. It must be remembered that other elements besides heredity should be taken into consideration when searching for evidence as to the inheritance of eczema. Members of families are apt to be under the same influences of diet, hygiene, etc., as well as exposed to the same atmospheric and other irritants, and this as well as any other disease may be developed in each individual, *de novo*, quite independent of any relations which they bear to each other.

Occasionally eczema will be found in connection with other skin affections, either existing at the same time, or developing the one upon the other. The following table shows that this was observed in about eight per cent. of the private cases. No notice is taken of skin diseases which may have preceded, but only those actually occurring under observation.

TABLE VI.—OTHER ERUPTIONS IN 1,200 PRIVATE PATIENTS.

DISEASES.	MALE.	FEMALE.	TOTAL.
Abscessus....................................	1		1
Acne	6	17	23
Alopecia....................................	4	2	6
Anthrax.....................................	2	1	3
Carcinoma..................................		1	1
Chloasma...................................	1	1	2
Dermatitis..................................	4		4
Epithelioma................................	2	1	3
Erysipelas..................................	1		1
Furunculi	9	8	17
Herpes......................................	9	1	10
Hyperidrosis................................	2	1	3
Ichthyosis..................................	1		1
Keloid......................................	1		1
Lichen......................................	2	2	4
Lupus......................................	1		1
Nævus pigmentosus..........................	1		1
Pemphigus..................................		1	1
Phthiriasis..................................	2	3	5
Pruritus....................................	1	2	3
Psoriasis...................................	9	6	15
Purpura....................................	1		1
Scabies.....................................	1		1
Syphilis....................................	4	2	6
Tinea trichophytina	6		6
Tinea versicolor	4		4
Ulcus	1		1
Urticaria...................................	1	1	2
Verruca....................................	1	1	2
Xanthoma		1	1
Xeroderma..................................	2		2
	80	52	132

It will be noticed that psoriasis and eczema were found thus connected in fifteen patients, while twenty-three cases presented, with the eczema an acne to a degree which called for medical intervention.

Furuncles and carbuncles, as also inflammation of the meibomian glands, are very common occurrences in eczema patients, and their frequency is by no means indicated in this table ; preceding the eczema, or happening during the course of treatment, they continually escaped record. No real relation can be established between them and the eruption ; sometimes it follows close upon one of these suppurative affections, and sometimes they come toward what proves to be the end of an obstinate eczema. Axillary abscesses are frequent in eczema of this region.

It would be a matter of considerable interest to develop the subject of the relationship of eczema to other diseases by means of statistics, but unfortunately records of these matters have not been kept to a sufficient degree of fullness, or with enough uniformity ; the material from which these statistics are drawn was not made for such a purpose as the present, but represents simply the records of disease taken at the time, dating fifteen years back, and entered solely for the purpose of thoroughly studying the cases with a view to treatment. It may be readily understood, therefore, that it would be almost impossible to record the relations of eczema to other diseases completely, even if the statements of patients could be always relied on.

It may not be without interest, however, to briefly state some points developed from a very considerable number of records among the private patients.

Malaria has been claimed to be a prolific source of eczema, as indeed of many other maladies. During the last five years I have made special inquiries of a large number of patients, and find that the malarial element counts for very little ; indeed, I have been surprised at the small proportion of those who give a malarial history. Many of these patients with eczema come from distant points, where malaria is entirely unknown, and comparatively few live in profoundly malarious districts.

Asthma has presented itself to me so frequently in connection with eczema, either in the persons affected or their immediate family, that I have come to look upon the complex state called asthma as in many instances but a condition of the pulmonary mucous tract similar to that found on the skin in eczema. Numbers of cases could be cited where the asthma alternated with attacks of eczema, and where, under prolonged and careful treatment for the eczema, the lung difficulty ceased.

Gout, or the gouty state, in the patient or immediate family, has also obtruded itself continually in my notes, and, as will be shown in another chapter, forms an important feature in the clinical study of eczema.

Rheumatism does not often appear thus associated, and stands in a very different relation to eczema, perhaps not occurring more frequently than many other diseases which do not suggest themselves as related to that under consideration.

Kidney disease, as such, is not associated with eczema as much as might be expected, considering the intimate physiological relations between the skin and kidneys. I have made and had made many hundreds of examinations of the urine of eczema patients, and albumen and casts have been found only as rarities, and sugar is very seldom seen.

But very few, indeed hardly any proportion, of those affected with eczema have suffered from severe kidney disorder, and among the entire number of patients, I believe that I do not know of any one dying from renal diseases. Nor are these met with in those closely related to eczema patients any more frequently than might naturally be expected; although the history is constantly given of near relations suffering from urinary derangements, gravel and stone; and these latter also have been more than naturally common among the eczema patients.

Functional disorder of the urinary secretion is very commonly met with, as will appear in another chapter, and its study is of value and interest in the management of eczema.

Liver difficulties—that is, functional derangements of this organ—are also of most frequent occurrence among eczema patients and their relatives, and will be more fully touched on later. Jaundice was not at all frequently met with, indeed almost never; and xanthelasma was rarely seen.

Lung diseases cannot be said to be associated with eczema in any important manner, although among a certain class of eczema cases in strumous subjects, the history of phthisis in the family is not at all uncommon. But, on the other hand, patients with eczema are as a rule free from lung trouble; except the asthmatic complications before alluded to. Nor do they acquire it when the eczema is removed.

Organic disease of the heart was rarely encountered, although many patients exhibited functional derangements, palpitation, irregularities of pulse, pain, etc., associated with dyspepsia, and often from the abuse of tobacco.

Serious nervous diseases were seldom seen, and no direct connection was noted between them and eczema. But neurasthenia and functional nervous symptoms were constantly observed, and often played a very important part in the genesis and prolongation of the disease, as will be more completely developed in other chapters.

CHAPTER III.

ECZEMA has been defined in a previous chapter as an inflammatory disease of the skin, of constitutional origin, manifesting various lesions and attended with itching or sensations referable to the nervous system. The earliest local phenomena were stated to be nerve and capillary disturbance, and the skin lesions were spoken of as secondary to these. We will now study in detail the features which eczema presents, and consider them in the order of their importance, which happens to be also the order of their pathological sequence. They may be arranged under six heads, which represent in a measure stages in the development of the local disease, as follows:

1. Itching, pricking, or burning pain.
2. Redness from congestion.
3. Papules, vesicles, pustules, or exudation.
4. Crusting, or scaling.
5. Infiltration or thickening.
6. Fissures or cracks.

It is essential that these phenomena should be well understood and remembered, both for a prompt recognition of the disease, and for the determining of the proper treatment.

1. Itching.—The most prominent and constant symptom in eczema is the itching, which may be preceded by, or give place to a burning pain, either of which are distressing beyond description. Those who have not suffered

from the itching of eczema can hardly appreciate any description of it.   When it is marked and severe, the desire
to scratch is simply irresistible, that is, in most instances,
and the injunction not to scratch a part affected greatly
with eczema is well-nigh useless without the assistance of
medical relief or physical restraint.   In some locations,
and in milder degrees of the complaint, the itching
amounts only to a disagreeable tickling or pricking, as
though a minute insect were irritating a nerve beneath
the skin, causing the patient to touch the part repeatedly;
while in other cases the sensation is that of insupportable
irritation or itching, which nothing will allay but the most
severe, deep, and thorough scratching or rubbing.   Between these two extremes all degrees of annoyance may
be experienced, and the sufferers seek various means of
allaying the irritation; for the lighter degrees of itching,
light touching, or tapping the part, or knocking it with
the knuckles suffices, or pinching it, as when a soft part
such as the scrotum is affected; more severe itching calls
forth moderate scratching, or rasping the part as with a
coarse towel; whereas, in long seated disease where there
is much infiltration, the itching is simply intolerable, and
only the most severe measures, as digging the skin with
the finger-nails, or even with a sharp instrument, etc.,
suffices to give relief.

I have placed this symptom of itching first and dwelt
upon it in order to impress the very great importance of
this element as a cause of many of the lesions of eczema,
and to emphasize its share in perpetuating the eruption.
It will often appear to be the sole trouble at first, and a
portion of the skin which had every external appearance
of health will itch, be torn with scratching, and the
severest eczema develop thereon.   Often, also, the itching will remain to a greater or less degree after the skin
lesions have been removed by treatment.   This itching is

always much worse when the part is exposed to the air, and the time of the greatest scratching of the parts of the body covered with clothing is on undressing at night, and on rising from the bed in the morning. In many portions the itching may come on with the slightest external irritation, and in many instances no adequate cause can be found for the paroxysms.

2. **Redness.**—The next most constant and striking symptom of eczema is the redness, without which the disease may be said not to exist. This redness is seen to be congestive, it disappearing almost if not quite entirely on pressure. In long standing erythematous eczema there remains a certain amount of reddish yellow staining after the blood has been forced out by pressure, caused by a previous escape of the coloring matter of the blood into the tissues, from the long continued capillary congestion. In some cases or forms of eczema this redness might be said to be the main objective feature, in addition to the itching and infiltration, the eruption remaining from first to last as an erythematous affection. This is seen most typically about the face, where we may have a surface of greater or less extent of a purplish red color, dry, harsh to the feel, sometimes shiny and sometimes covered with a moderate amount of thin scales. This erythematous surface, however, has the deep tingling, itching, or burning characteristic of eczema; it is chronic, that is, instead of coming quickly and spreading rapidly as would erythema or erysipelas, it develops slowly and is not attended with any febrile disturbance; and, finally, it has an element characteristic of eczema in the thickening of the skin, which will be described later as a most constant and marked symptom of the eruption.

3. **Papules, Vesicles, Pustules, or Exudation.**—From what has been said of the nature of the process in eczema, it can be readily understood what part these surface

lesions play in the disease. Eczema being an inflammatory eruption of the catarrhal type, the exudation from the congested vessels seeks to gain exit from the meshes of the skin where it finds itself. When the congestion is more especially around the follicles, the plastic fluid which is poured out forms small solid papules, very red, pointed, and itchy. If the fluid is more abundant and less plastic it raises the epidermis, and vesicles are formed; or, pustules are formed if there is a great intensity of inflammation, or a lowered state of vitality, or a strumous habit. When, however, the surface is broken, as after the formation and rupture of vesicles and pustules, the fluid exudes directly from the surface and forms the "watering," "leeting," or discharging surface very commonly seen. In some cases this exudative or sweating stage occurs apparently without the previous existence of the intermediate one of vesicles or pustules. The epidermis seems to be lifted in a mass by the abundance of the watery discharge, and this raw surface will be seen very soon after the congestive stage has appeared. Such a condition is frequently observed in places where the skin is very delicate and kept moist, as in the folds about the genitals, beneath the mammæ, and around the necks of children.

This constant tendency to exude fluid from the capillaries is a striking and common feature of eczema, and one which is intimately dependent upon the nature of the disease, and is closely connected with its pathology.

4. **Crusting and Scaling.**—The exudate of eczema, which has the property of stiffening and staining linen, has a very strong tendency to dry into crusts and scales if exposed to the air. Take an ordinary discharging eczematous surface and leave it uncovered for a while, and it will first be seen to become glazed over, and the finger touched to it will no longer perceive the previous sticky condition, but all is dry and slippery. A little later this

film increases from beneath, and there is a coating of varying thickness, which may reach the formation of considerable masses.   Especially is this the case in pustular eczema, and in the eruption in infants we sometimes see large and thick collections of dried exudation, which when matted in the hair are very difficult of removal ; beneath these crusts the surface is found still moist and exuding, and if the masses are removed by washing, or are forcibly torn off, the exudation will again and again form a similar coating of dried matter.   If the surface has been scratched, blood may be mingled with the exudate, and the crusts will be of a dark color.   Upon those regions of the body where the sebaceous glands are large and numerous, as on the scalp and bearded face, there is always a considerable sebaceous element mixed with the exudate of the eczema.   The disease process seems to extend into the cavity of the glands, and to both increase the quantity and alter the quality of the secretion ; the crusts may then be more yellow, and gummy, and tenacious in larger masses.   If the exudation is not excessive, in place of the crusts there are only scales of varying thickness.   Not at all infrequently on the legs we have a red, shiny surface covered to a greater or less degree with scaly crusts, which adhere until forcibly dislodged ; when removed they will sometimes come off in large masses, and leave a slightly moist surface beneath, which will again coat itself in a short time with a similar formation.

Still another condition of scaliness is seen where there never has been any moist element whatever ; but the erythematous surface simply sheds its epidermal coat repeatedly in larger or smaller scales.   Such a condition is very common on the scalp, and forms many of the cases which pass under the general name of "dandruff."

5. **Infiltration or Thickening.**—Skin which has been for some time the seat of the eczematous process ac-

quires a feature which is of the greatest importance both diagnostically and therapeutically; this is what is known as infiltration or thickening, and is an essential element of the chronic forms of the eruption, and closely dependent upon its nature. Eczema has been thus far described as a catarrhal inflammation of the skin, and it is this discharge feature which produces many of the clinical phenomena. The fluid which exudes from the vessels, with a certain number of leucocytes, is poured out first into the deeper structures of the skin about the capillaries. If the amount is not too large, it is retained in the meshes of the corium and first causes some œdema; or, becoming organized, it produces the infiltration or thickening. The disease process may become arrested at this stage, and either retrograde, with absorption of the effused products, or it may remain in this condition indefinitely, the infiltration remaining constant or increasing, and a chronic erythematous eczema result. This infiltration is an element in all long standing cases of eczema, and becomes then the main object for treatment, for upon its presence depends much of the itching, the scaling, and, if the surface is irritated, the exudation. In certain instances this infiltration, which at first involves the rete mucosum and papillary layer, may extend through the entire structure of the derma, and affect even the panniculus adiposus, and the resulting thickening of the skin may be so great as to cause it to appear firmly attached to the subjacent parts. It is recognized clinically by the increased thickness of a fold of integument when pinched up between the fingers and compared with a corresponding portion of unaffected skin. The great clinical importance of this symptom is that while this thickening remains the eczema is not cured, but will pretty certainly return when treatment is suspended, even though the surface may appear smooth and free from scales or evidence of disease.

In some instances this infiltration becomes so great that the structures take on an hypertrophic condition, and a leg and foot especially may present an appearance very closely resembling elephantiasis Arabum ; but this may all be made entirely to disappear by sufficient and proper treatment, and is only a magnified condition of what is ordinarily seen.

6. **Fissures or Cracks.**—Closely connected with the infiltration is another feature of eczema, which demands careful attention and often proves very rebellious, namely, the formation of fissures or cracks in the skin; these are, as a rule, exceedingly painful, and at times quite incapacitate those suffering from them.   This cracking of the skin is indeed dependent upon the last symptom mentioned, namely, the infiltration, and is found where the tissue, which has thus lost its normal suppleness, is called upon to stretch and bend.   The infiltration of the whole texture of the skin with the products of inflammation, renders the fibres, which should be elastic in the highest degree, dense and hard; and the presence of the inflammatory cells, without cohesive power, in and among the fibres of the derma weakens what strength is left, and every movement tears into the tender and sensitive corium bereft of its epidermis.

These fissures are seen in their greatest severity on the hands, both on the knuckles and in the palm; they are also found behind the ears, at the bends of the knees and elbows, indeed in any location where there is motion. They are not, however, characteristic of eczema alone, for they are seen in syphilis of the palm and elsewhere, also occasionally in psoriasis, etc.   These fissures need not always be in the lines of motion ; often on the palms they occur in any direction.

The inflammatory process of acute eczema does not appear to differ from that which takes place in ordinary

inflammation of the skin of purely local origin, or dermatitis, and inasmuch as this latter can be produced at will
on the lower animals, we can there study the phenomena
from the beginning. For this purpose Neumann rubbed
croton oil upon the ear of a white rabbit for ten or fifteen
minutes, and then watched the result through a microscope of low power for several hours. Rhythmical contraction of the vessels first took place, they being at one
moment full of blood, and empty at the next; later, they
became permanently dilated and stasis took place. The
ear which before was translucent became cloudy, swollen,
and hot, and in a few hours numerous vesicles appeared
with serous contents. After forty-eight hours the animal
was killed and the tissue was found soaked with a serous
fluid and the cutis infiltrated with a large number of cells.

Biesiadecki has described the condition found in papules and vesicles taken from true idiopathic eczema.
The papillæ are enlarged by infiltration with serous fluid
and cells, and their connective tissue corpuscles are increased in number and size and are very succulent. There
also appear numerous spindle-shaped cells reaching from
the papillæ between the cells of rete malpighii which they
crowd apart. As the exudation increases from the capillaries the fluid penetrates the papillæ along these chan-
nels or ways which have been made, and accumulates to
form a vesicle. The papule is formed by the infiltration
of a group of papillæ. More recent investigations by
Gaucher have shown that the cells of the rete malpighii
also probably take an active part in the process of eczema, and that vacuoles are formed within it, apparently from
a distension of individual cells with fluid; these uniting
form vesicles, or if they are very abundant the epidermal
surface is stripped off by the fluid.

The fluid which escapes from idiopathic eczema has
been examined and is found to be composed of serum

containing leucocytes, and as far as can be determined differs in no way from that contained in an ordinary blister artificially produced. I have sometimes found the fluid neutral, sometimes alkaline.

The pathology of chronic eczema has also been studied by a number of observers (Neumann, Rindfleisch, Kaposi, Riemer), and the conditions found by all agree very closely. Here we have the *results* of the preceding inflammatory process, seen in enlarged papillæ and diffuse cell infiltration.

In long standing eczema the papillæ become so greatly enlarged as to be visible in some cases to the naked eye. This can be best observed on the legs in an old case of red and moist eczema. The diseased part should be freed from scales and have a tendency to exude, and if closely examined the surface will appear as if a fine gauze was stretched over it, the spaces between the meshes being of a deeper red, while the net-work is of a decidedly whitish hue. The red points are the enlarged papillæ and the mesh-work is the deeper portion of the malpighian layer, rightly called the rete mucosum, or mucous net, here shown as it dips down around each papilla.

This infiltration of the skin in old cases of eczema may extend even to involving the entire structure of the integument, including the adipose tissue, and observers describe great cell and pigment deposit especially about the dilated blood-vessels; a dilatation of the lymphatics; hardening of the connective tissue; destruction of the sebaceous glands and hair follicles; degeneration of the sweat glands and disappearance of the fat cells; in short, the changes seen in degenerative hypertrophy, as in elephantiasis Arabum, have all been observed in chronic eczema. In one case recently described by Pasquet, the degeneration went so far as to destroy the nails completely and to convert the ends of the fingers into useless stumps.

Many of the phenomena of eczema point strongly to nerve relations of the eruption, and the recognition of these is of the greatest importance to the full understanding of the disease under consideration. This subject will be more fully developed clinically in the chapter on the causes of eczema, but the anatomical portion of it may be best considered here.

It must be borne well in mind that the nervous supply of the skin is enormous, so great and so evenly distributed that the finest needle cannot enter the surface without causing pain. Until quite recently it was supposed that the nerve distribution was confined entirely to the corium, and terminated externally within the papillæ, in certain bodies called the tactile corpuscles. Microscopic researches during the last ten years have demonstrated that certain nerve fibres, after running a short distance beneath the mucous layer, enter among its cells; others after reaching the papilla, subdivide within it, and leaving it penetrate between the cells of the rete malpighii. In favorable specimens the nerve-fibres are readily seen entering the mucous layer and ending there in knob-like distensions, at the height, perhaps, of the third row of cells. Also in the more external layers of the rete, Langerhans asserts that he has seen a number of bodies, stained violet in chloride of gold, which he thinks are connected with deeper nerve fibres, sending prolongations downwards and several outwards in the direction of horny layer. Others have verified the presence of these non-medullated fibres among the epithelial layers of the skin in lower animals, and they have also been followed among the epithelial cells lining the sebaceous glands.

The nervous connection and relations in eczema can also be traced from a pathological point of view, as regards this and other affections of the skin. Thus, the dependence of certain skin lesions upon nerve states or alterations is now decided beyond controversy. The most striking instance is in the case of zoster, where the erythema and vesiculation of the skin is directly dependent upon nerve inflammation, seated chiefly in the ganglion located on the posterior or sensitive root of the spinal nerves. The number of post-mortem examinations which have shown nerve inflammation in zoster is now very considerable, and the results reported have been very uniform. Besides zoster, many other lesions on the skin have been traced to nerve origin, as, the skin changes seen to follow injuries of nerves, which need not be mentioned here; this subject was fully studied by the writer in a number of articles, to which reference must be made for further proof of this point.*

In regard to the mode in which the nerve element comes into play in the production of the lesions of eczema, there are several ways in which they may be produced. First, through the direct agency of the nerve influence. In the same manner in which the cells of a part, under normal nerve influence, appropriate just sufficient nutriment to insure their healthy condition, and in turn yield up their effete elements in a healthy manner, so under perverted innervation the cells take on the phenomena which we know as inflammation. While the existence of proper trophic nerves has not yet been demonstrated microscopically, there cannot be the slightest doubt but that nerve influence can and does preside over good or bad nutrition. Second: the results are claimed by some to be brought about through the influence of the capillary system, the vaso-motor nerves acting to produce a contraction and dilatation of the finer blood-vessels, as previously described in simple dermatitis, which results finally in sta-

* Archives of Electrology and Neurology, Nov. 1874, May, 1875. Chicago Journal of Nervous and Mental Disease, October, 1875. Amer. Jour. Med. Sciences, July, 1876.

sis; the exudation of serum and the escape of leucocytes being secondary to this. Third: many of the lesions of eczema can be accounted for by the scratching, or by the irritation given to the skin by measures employed for the relief of the itching. None of these explanations suffices alone to explain all the phenomena of eczema, but they are all of importance to remember in the practical management of the disease, as will appear hereafter. Here our anatomical studies merge into clinical, and the remainder of this subject will be discussed in a subsequent chapter in connection with other causes of eczema.

CHAPTER IV.

FORMS OF ECZEMA.—ACUTE, SUB-ACUTE, AND CHRONIC.

No little confusion has arisen in regard to recognizing and managing eczema from the multitude of names
which from time to time have been given to the different
manifestations or phases of the eruption. It has so often
been attempted to explain the special character, or location, or condition of the eruption by the name given to it,
that the nomenclature of this single disease has become so
vast that it is perplexing to the general practitioner, and
annoying even to those who have much to do with this
branch. Thus, in the index of Mr. Wilson's "Lectures on
Ekzema," there are forty-nine varieties found, not as syn-
onyms, but each is treated of separately in the work; and,
in the index of McCall Anderson's Treatise on Eczema,
forty-three distinct names occur, and thirty-four in the
index of Duhring's work. I have made a collection
of the terms thus employed in these and many other
books, and although the list is probably not complete, it is
found that not less than one hundred and twenty-five
Latin names have been given to the phases of this one
eruption, while the total number of terms collected, including those in more common use in English, French,
and German, amounts to nearly one hundred and eighty!

But an analysis of these names shows that they may
mostly be grouped in a few classes, and have been devised
to express certain points in reference to the eruption;
while a certain number relate to fanciful features or are

popular terms in different languages. Now, although these prominent features which it has been attempted to express in the name of the eruption are, in the main, real and of importance to an understanding of the disease, still, unless the subject is looked at clearly and understood properly, the mass of terms applied to eczema becomes exceedingly confusing. Herewith are given the names, grouped as far as possible in five classes, while those which do not permit of such grouping, often from the wrong application of the name in former times, are thrown into a sixth, miscellaneous class. The classes are as follows:

1st. Relating to the Stage of the eruption; as, Acute, Chronic, etc.

2d. According to the Lesion present; Papular, Vesicular, etc.

3d. Expressing the Condition; as Crusted, Fissured, Moist, etc.

4th. Indicating Causes; as, Artificial, Scrofulous, Hereditary, Infantile, etc.

5th. Designating the Location; as, of the Face, Hands, Feet, etc.

6th. Miscellaneous.

Names given to eczema in the literature of Dermatology, together with synonymes :

1. Stages.	Eczema acutum :—sub-acutum :—chronicum :—simplex :—compositum :—vulgaris :—fugax :—perstans :—inveteratum :—mite :—succesivum (recurrent).
2. Lesion.	Eczema erythematosum (erythematodes or erythematous) :—papulosum (papular) :—vesiculosum (vesicular) :—pustulosum (pustular).
3. Condition.	Eczema amorphe :—circumscriptum :—coriaceum :—crustaceum : —crustosum :—exanthematosum :—exfoliativum :—fendillé :—figuratum :—fissum :—foliaceum :—furfuraceum :—herpetiforme .—humidum :—ichorosum (ichorous) :—impetiginosum :—impetigi-

nodes (impetiginous) : — intertrigo : — lichenoides (lichenous) :—
madidans :—marginatum :—mucosum :—nummulare :—œdemato-
sum :—pityriasicum :—psoriasiforme :—rimosum :—rubrum:—sic-
cum : — sclerosum (sklerosum) : — spargosiforme : — squamosum
(squamous) : —sycosiforme : — tuberosum : — unisquamosum :—
verrucosum.

4. Causes.   Eczema arthriticum (arthritique) : artificial : assimilative :
caloricum : congenital :—dartreux : hereditary :—herpetique :
—infantile :—mercuriale (hydrargyria) :—neurosum (neurotic):
nutritive :—scrofuleux :—solare : substitutive : traumatic: varicose.

5 Location.   Eczema ani :—articulorum ·—aurium :—axillarum :—barbæ (pilare
faciei) :—capillitii :—capitis :—corporis :—crurale (crurum) :—dif-
usum :—digitorum :—dorsi manûs :—extremitatum :—faciei : —
genitale (genitalium) :—inguinum :—labiorum :—mammæ (mam-
marum) :—mammillarum :—manuum :—narium :—oris et labiorum :—partiale :—palmare et plantare :—palpebrarum : —pedum :
penis :—perinæi : — pudendi :—tarsi :—trunci :—umbilici :—um-
bilicale :—unguium :—universale (general).

6. Miscellaneous.   Baker's itch : barber's itch : bricklayer's itch : grocer's itch :
washerwoman's itch : crusta lactea : cytisma eczema : ecphly-
sis : dartre crustacée flavescente : dartre crustacée stalactiforme :
dartre squameuse humide : dartre squameuse orbiculaire : dartre
vive : eczema sudorale : eczesis : eczesma : eczesmus : fluxus
salinus : heat eruption : herpes squamosus madidans : hitz-
blätterchen : humid scall : humid tetter : impetigo : impetigo
acniforme : impetigo eczematodes : impetigo erysipelatodes :
impetigo figurata : impetigo scabida : impetigo sparsa : impetigo
sycosiforme : lichen agrius : lichen hypertrophique : lichen tropi-
cus : melitagra : melitagra flavescens : mentagra : milk crust :
nässende flechte : porrigine amiantacée : porrigo crustacea : porrigo larvalis : poussée : psoriasis diffusa : red gum : running scall :
salt rheum : scabies humida : scall : sycosis : teigne furfuracée :
tinea amientacea : tinea asbestina : tinea granulata (teigne gran-
ulée) : tinea micacea : tinea mucosa (teigne muquese) : tooth
rash.

Many of the terms in this list are now entirely obsolete
and many have never been accepted by others than those
proposing them, but a large number are of value and are
still used at times. But if the plan and object of the
names are kept in view their number need not give difficulty. It must be remembered that in every instance the
disease is the same, and the names are only given to indicate differences in the appearance, condition, or location

of the lesion, so that the same eruption may receive a name taken from each of these six classes to distinguish features belonging to it. Thus, an acute pustular eczema of the face in a strumous child might be spoken of as eczema (1) acutum, (2) pustulosum, (3) crustosum, (4) scrofulosum, (5) faciei, and in older writings would be described under the name (6) impetigo figurata, or would now often be spoken of as milk crust; or, a chronic eczema of the hands with cracks, in a washerwoman could have the name, eczema (1) chronicum, (2) papulosum, (3) fissum, (4) artificiale, (5) manuum, and might be popularly called (6) washerwoman's itch.

Understanding then the meaning and the application of the various terms used in connection with eczema, we find that there are comparatively few which need be employed ordinarily. But the five classes which form the basis of the nomenclature should be remembered; there are features pertaining to each which are of constant use in treating of the subject, and are here employed. First, then, we divide eczema according to its stages, as follows:

1. Stages,	acute	eczema acutum.
	sub-acute	" sub-acutum.
	chronic	" chronicum.

Next every case may be classed according to the predominant lesion, or the form of the eruption:

2. Predominant lesion,	erythematous	eczema erythematosum.
	papular	" papulosum.
	vesicular	" vesiculosum.
	pustular	" pustulosum.

Then it is often of service to indicate the condition generally present, which often represents secondary lesions, or results of disease. There are many designations thus used, such as the following:

3. Condition,	moist	eczema madidans or rubrum.
	scaly	" squamosum or exfoliativum.
	hard	" sclerosum.
	fissured	" fissum or rimosum.

To express the cause of the eczema we have also a number of names which are of service:

CONSTITUTIONAL.

	gouty	eczema arthriticum.	
	strumous	" strumosum.	
	neurotic	" neuroticum.	
4. Cause,		LOCAL.	
	traumatic	eczema traumaticum.	
	varicose	" e varices.	
	artificial	" artificiale.	

In addition to the names of the various portions of the body which may be added in Latin to designate the location, there are several others which are at times of service, such as the following:

5. Location,	diffuse	eczema diffusum.	
	partial	" partiale.	
	universal	" universale.	

Finally there are certain of the popular terms which have been and will long be applied to the various manifestations of eczema, such as crusta lactea or milk crust; baker's, bricklayer's, grocer's, and washerwoman's itch; tooth rash; heat eruption; red gum; also others in French and German. These will pass out of use as greater enlightenment prevails on the subject of diseases of the skin.

It will thus be seen that the form of eczema, or exactly the name to be given to the manifestation in any particular case is not a matter of the very greatest importance, for the same eruption may receive a different name at one or another period of its course, or to indicate one or another feature. It is well, however, to be able to fix in the mind certain prominent points bearing upon each case, and these may be briefly touched upon.

The first point, and a most important one to be taken into consideration in connection with the diagnosis and also the treatment of eczema, is the stage or state of the existing eruption. By this is understood, not so much the length of time which the disease has lasted, as the condition in which the skin is found as regards the intensity of the inflammatory process; for cases of eczema exhibit the most marked differences according to the stage, condition, or variety of the eruption.

Three stages or general states may be spoken of, acute, sub-acute, and chronic; an acute eczematous condition of skin may develop in a case which has lasted for many years, or a sub-acute state may remain for a long period, ever ready to manifest acute symptoms with undue irritation, or to subside into a chronic condition if undisturbed or under soothing treatment.

Acute eczema is characterized by heat, burning and tingling of the skin, with redness and œdema, which latter may be very considerable, especially in regions where the skin is lax, as about the face, penis, etc. Shortly papules and vesicles appear, or even pustules, or the surface may remain evenly red, and occasionally have the epidermis stripped off quickly, leaving a raw, exuding surface. Vesicles belong to acute eczema, but are by no means always seen in it; sometimes, especially on the hands, they occur in immense numbers, and thickly set together. They are also seen in sub-acute eczema, though comparatively rarely, and most seldom in the real chronic form. The term acute eczema is applied both to first attacks and to recurrences or sharp exacerbations of the eruption in old cases. Acute eczema often resembles artificial eruptions very closely, and it may be very difficult, if not impossible to distinguish at once between an attack of acute eczema and the eruption excited by poison ivy, poisonous dyes, as in socks, or even an eruption produced by arnica, croton oil, etc.

If the eruption of acute eczema is protected, or not further irritated, it will tend to subside in a few days, but it has little if any tendency to disappear entirely; some of the elements of the eruption linger and either there are recurrences of the acute symptoms, or, as occurs more commonly, it lapses into a less active condition and passes into the next state.

Sub-acute eczema represents a less inflammatory condition, generally presenting a reddened, itchy surface, with moderate thickening, which may be either moist, tending to cover itself with crusts and scales, or may be studded with papules which give exit to a glairy fluid whenever they are torn by scratching; this latter is often the case on account of the intense itching which generally accompanies this form of eruption. Under irritating local agencies or certain deranged internal states, as constipation, severe dyspepsia, etc., this may be lighted up into an acute eruption, or, under favoring circumstances it tends to subside into the next form.

Chronic eczema exhibits very many different states or conditions of disease, from a diffusely reddened and thickened skin, covering possibly the whole body, and itching furiously and desquamating freely, to a single, small patch of diseased tissue, thickened and hard, tending to crack when exposed to motion, and having a deep, intolerable sensation of itching or tickling, which it seems almost impossible to relieve, except by the severest and deepest digging and scratching. The lines of demarcation betwen acute, sub-acute and chronic eczema are not sharply defined, but it is important to remember all the phases of the eruption in diagnosis, and especially important to appreciate them in reference to treatment, as will be pointed out later.

The next item to be considered is the form which the eruption takes in regard to its predominant anatomical lesion; and here we find four quite distinct conditions.

Eczema erythematosum, erythematous eczema. This is marked from first to last, by the erythema-like character of its lesion ; appearing first as a redness of greater or less extent and degree, with some œdema, the surface maintains this as a striking feature to the end. Some infiltration may always be made out, and a certain amount of fine desquamation, and there is a peculiar hard leathery feel, and an absence of the normal unctuous condition, owing to interference with the action of the sebaceous glands. There is always the deep pricking, tingling, burning, or tickling sensation, which is often exceedingly distressing.

The degree and extent of the redness are subject to great variations, both in different cases and in the same individual at different times and conditions. It may be almost absent for a while, and only the deep tickling remain ; or it may cover a considerable surface and be of a bright red color. Sometimes it is almost of a purple tint, or an old erythematous eczema may acquire a yellowish, leathery hue. All agents which excite the circulation, such as exercise, liquor, sudden change of temperature, etc., will cause patches of erythematous eczema, about the face especially, to acquire a brilliant color, while under cooling measures, external and internal, it can pale greatly. It is apt to be a very chronic affair, and about the face and head generally causes much annoyance or even distress : this is often wrongly called *chronic erysipelas.*

Eczema papulosum, or papular eczema. In this form the congestion and exudation are localized and circumscribed, and hard, red, inflammatory, acuminated papules are formed, appearing quickly and tending to remain for some time, days or even weeks. They may be isolated, or grouped together upon a reddened base, and are generally seen to be scratched and torn, for the itching accompanying this form is usually excessive.

Typical papular eczema may run its course from first to last with papules as its only lesion, but very commonly small vesicles appear, and even pustules, and there is always more or less of erythematous eczema between. Much that was called lichen by older writers is now recognized as papular eczema.

Eczema vesiculosum, vesicular eczema.   While eczema was formerly described as a vesicular eruption, it is acknowledged to-day that the vesicle is not a necessary lesion in any particular case ; moreover, true and typical eczema vesiculosum, in which all or a majority of the lesions are vesicles, is comparatively rare, although a little care may detect vesicles in many cases.

Typical vesicular eczema is usually an acute affair ; there is a feeling of heat and tension about a part, with some œdema, and very soon minute red points are seen which quickly vesiculate, and within a few hours there may be a considerable crop of vesicles of some size ; they are generally in groups and frequently run together, making a patch. The burning and itching, which is sometimes very intense, is very greatly lessened or even ceases when the fluid has reached the surface in the vesicles, and especially when these are ruptured and it escapes. If the surface is undisturbed by scratching, and appropriate treatment is employed, the vesicles may subside without rupture and the acute attack cease, and be followed by desquamation.   More commonly the vesicles are broken and the exuded fluid tends to form crusts ; or, a weeping, red surface may result, the eczema rubrum or madidans, and the amount of fluid exuded from such a surface is sometimes very great.

Very frequently the vesicular stage is of such short duration that the single elements of it escape notice, and the case is first seen with a moist, exuding surface, or with one covered with scales or crusts, as especially occurs in eczema in infants and children.

If the inflammation runs very high, or if there is a low

state of vitality, or a strumous condition, the vesicles soon tend to pass into pustules.

Eczema pustulosum, pustular eczema, known also as impetiginous eczema, or eczema impetiginosum or impetiginodes. The lines of separation between this and the preceding variety or form of eruption are not well marked, although typical cases of the two present quite distinct features. The mode of development and formation of the lesions are much the same in both, the difference appears to be mainly in the lowered vitality which causes the production of pus in the latter, in place of more active inflammatory products. There is usually very much less itching in this than in other forms of the eruption. As in vesicular eczema the vesicles may not be observed, so often pustular eczema is brought for treatment presenting only light or dark greenish-yellow crusts, which when occurring upon hairy parts, a favorite seat, may mat the hairs together in an almost inextricable mass: upon the hairy face the pustules are often very distinct and remain intact for some time.

It will be understood that in thus attempting to describe the different conditions or forms in which we find eczema it is by no means intimated that these features are sharply cut; they often merge into each other, and often the face of the eruption is so altered that it is difficult to say positively what was originally the predominant primary lesion. This brings us to the consideration of the next phases which the eruption may exhibit, and based upon which certain names have been given to the eruption, as it is presented clinically.

The third division of the names which have been applied to eczema, therefore relates to what may be spoken of as the condition of the eruption; here there are a large number of terms which explain themselves, some of which are of more or less value, and, being in constant use, they are often employed to represent forms of the eruption. As the preceding four varieties represent primary lesions or the modes of development of the eruption, so these are to be regarded as secondary conditions, depending upon a previous pathological process. A few of the more commonly used terms will receive attention.

Eczema madidans, or rubrum, results from a shedding of the epidermis and the exposure of a diseased rete malpighii giving exit to serous exudation ; the extent of this varies very considerably. The most typical examples are found in old cases of eczema of the lower extremities, where the entire surface of one or both legs may be red, raw, painful, and exuding vast quantities of serum, which readily dries into crusts or scales, or stiffens and causes dressings to adhere to the part. The same condition is seen in the faces and heads of infants, where the surface is washed again and again, or where it is torn in the frantic efforts of the child to obtain relief from the itching; it also occurs in the flexures of the joints and where folds of skin are in contact.

Eczema squamosum, or squamous eczema, represents a secondary stage following any of the conditions which have been described. There is a continuous exfoliation of epidermis, generally from a reddened surface, which may represent the declining stage of the eruption, or may persist as an active element, as in the case of erythematous eczema, where the surface commonly presents scales almost from the first. Upon the scalp almost the entire disease from first to last may appear on superficial observation to be a free desquamation, constituting many cases of so-called "dandruff;" but here redness can also be found, with infiltration and itching, and generally some well marked eczema elsewhere.

Eczema sclerosum. Upon the palms and soles especially eczema sometimes takes the form simply of hardening and thickening of the integument, either in patches or covering the entire surface : there may be little or no desquamation, never any moisture, papules, or vesicles, but simply the thickened and leathery condition of the skin, generally accompanied with deep burning or itching. This condition has sometimes wrongly been spoken of as a scleroderma, but this term is applied to an entirely different affection ; a little close observation of these cases for some time will demonstrate their eczematous nature. A heightened degree of this hard condition has been described by certain writers under the name *eczema verrucosum ;* in this a small, circumscribed portion is hard and wart-like, perhaps with deep and painful fissures or cracks.

Eczema fissum or rimosum, eczema fendillé of the French. Closely allied to the last form of eczema, and dependent upon the infiltration, we find the fissuring of the skin, and sometimes as at the ends of the fingers the cracking will appear to be about the only element of disease. For these cases this term is peculiarly suitable.

Eczema infantile. No particular form or phase of eczema is indicated by this name, any or all the conditions previously described may be seen in infants, but on account of the many clinical features in its etiology and management, the designation is applied to cases of the disease occurring during the first five years of life ; many cases beginning during this period last for many years afterwards.

Of the remaining large number of names given on a preceding page, as having been applied to eczema, very many of them have but little importance at the present day ; as far as possible those which may be of service will be referred to in subsequent pages. If, therefore, information is desired in regard to them, it may often be obtained by consulting the index.

CHAPTER V.

DIAGNOSIS OF ECZEMA.—PROGNOSIS.

ECZEMA may resemble and be mistaken for very many of the diseases of the skin, and a correct diagnosis in every case is a feat of no slight difficulty to those unaccustomed to see many patients with affections of the skin: its protean appearances resemble now one and now another cutaneous lesion, in a manner often very puzzling. It should be stated, however, that more errors occur in supposing cases to be eczema which are not this eruption than in failing to recognize the disease when present. Although eczema is by far the most common of all affections of the skin, and, as has been shown, is exhibited by at least one third, perhaps one half, of all patients with skin diseases, yet the other half or two thirds of the cases is made up of so many different varieties of skin disorders that the practitioner finds himself far more prone to regard some other eruption eczema than he is to call a case of real eczema by another name.

Two methods of diagnosis may be employed; the one that of recognizing the disease by means of its own symptoms alone, and the other that of reaching the diagnosis by means of the exclusion of other eruptions from the absence of their proper symptoms; neither alone suffices, but both methods are required in deciding the character of an eruption, and in recognizing eczema. It is not only necessary to bear well in mind the actual characters of the disease, but one should also know and remember what other eruptions the one under consideration might be, and by recognizing the one and excluding the others a correct diagnosis can be arrived at with almost a perfect certainty.

The symptoms of eczema have been fully detailed in a preceding chapter and need not be dwelt upon largely here. It will be remembered that they were grouped under six headings; namely, 1. Itching, or burning pain: 2. Redness, from congestion: 3. Papules, vesicles, pustules, or exudation: 4. Crusting and scaling: 5. Infiltration or thickening of the skin: and 6. Fissures or cracks. In making the diagnosis these elements are to be sought for and recognized as far as possible. Generally most of them can be observed in each case of eczema some time during its course, although they may not all be present at once at any particular spot of eruption. The actual state of the skin varies very greatly according to the stage existing at the time of observation. Itching and redness are universal symptoms of eczema, but they of course pertain to other skin maladies as well; papules, vesicles, and pustules also occur in many other diseases. But the exudative character of eczema is a striking one, and if this symptom is present, or if there is a good history of the same, it aids the diagnosis greatly. The infiltration or thickening of the skin is another feature almost peculiar to eczema, although certain patches of lichen planus, also some large tracts of psoriasis may resemble eczema somewhat in this respect. The crusting and scaling of eczema are generally quite characteristic, and will be dwelt on later, as also the cracking.

The particular phases or appearances presented by the eruption on different parts of the body will be detailed and explained in connection with eczema of various localities, and the differential diagnosis in each case will be pointed out. At present the general features of diagnosis will be treated of, and the eruptions which may at times be mistaken for eczema will be described. Reference may be made to this chapter with advantage in connection with the diagnosis of the diseases in each locality.

As remarked before, the eruption of eczema may be mistaken for very many skin lesions, and I find that there are no less than twenty-eight other eruptions which are liable to be, and most of which I have seen confounded with the disease under consideration, even by physicians. It is unnecessary to enter here fully into every feature of all the eruptions which may resemble eczema, inasmuch as the special differences will be more fully dwelt on again in speaking of the management of the disease as it affects different portions of the body ; but brief mention will be made of them here in alphabetical order.

1. **Acne.**—The rosaceous form of acne, with small, hard papules on an erythematous base, seated especially about the cheeks or chin sometimes resembles eczema ; but as a rule a sebaceous element can be discovered in the former, moreover the itching which is very annoying in eczema of this region is almost if not entirely absent in acne, or is replaced by a burning, or by pain in the spots when pressed. Acne sebacea or seborrhœa about the nose is distinguished from eczema by the greasy character of the crusts and the absence of much redness and itching. On the scalp acne sebacea or seborrhœa is differentiated from chronic scaly eczema, also by the greasiness of the scales, and the absence of itching.

2. **Dermatitis.**—Simple inflammation of the skin, as from heat, poison ivy, etc., is often quite indistinguishable from eczema for a while, but the history of the case, the ready disappearance of the eruption on the removal of the cause, and the absence of exudation, infiltration, and itching later on, will readily distinguish between

the two. A dermatitis may be the starting point of a true eczema.

3. **Dysidrosis.**—This affection of the hands, named also cheiro-pompholyx and pompholyx, has small pearly, or sago-like vesicles on and between the fingers, which resemble greatly those of eczema, and considerable discussion has arisen in regard to the true nature of some of the cases thus reported. The lines of demarcation between the two eruptions are not sharply and certainly defined as yet; in the main, however, the vesicles of dysidrosis tend to remain discrete and to dry up soon, whereas eczema is prolonged, and attended with more inflammatory signs; both affections burn and itch considerably. An eczema will almost always appear elsewhere as well, or there will be a history which will clear up the diagnosis.

4. **Epithelioma.**—Well marked cases of this affection. with hard, everted edges and ulcerated base, should never suggest eczema, but I have seen a number of very mild cases early in their development which had been always previously regarded as eczema by the medical men who had seen them. These are characterized by a superficial degeneration of the outer layers of the skin, which dry down into a thin scaly crust, and when this is removed, as it constantly is by scratching, a slightly moist and generally a slightly bleeding surface remains, which soon becomes covered again with a similar thin crust, to be again picked off; there is now very little that can be called ulceration, and the edges are hardly if at all prominent. But the small and very localized character of the lesion, the sharply defined margins, as distinguished from the fading border of eczema, the absence of thickening and the very slight if any itching should be sufficient to separate it from eczema. These cases are generally seen on the face; commonly an eczema presenting any lesion at all resembling this, would show itself elsewhere as well.

The disease on the female nipples, and areolæ preceding
the development of carcinoma, which has been under discussion in England recently under the name of " so-called
eczema," is probably not an eczema at all, but a very early
manifestation of epithelial degeneration ; this will be more
particularly noticed in connection with eczema of the
trunk and breast.

  5. **Erysipelas.**—Many cases of erythematous eczema
are wrongly called erysipelas, but a careful study should
easily prevent such a mistake in diagnosis. Erysipelas
is an acute disease, accompanied by fever and constitutional disturbance; the inflammation of the skin is
intense, there is great heat of the part, and œdematous
swelling; the eruption spreads rapidly, with a burning sensation, and a fiery red, shining, and tense surface, and without the tendency to a discharge ; nor is there any scaling
until the acute febrile process is over. The erythematous
form of eczema, especially about the face, sometimes resembles this in a slight degree, but without the fever, constitutional disturbance, etc. ; moreover, there is itching and
some scaling, and thickening almost from the first.
There is of course no such thing as a chronic erysipelas,
as is sometimes spoken of in connection with these cases
of chronic erythematous eczema of the face and eczema
rubrum of the legs; in this latter location the discharge
and scaling are pathognomic.

  6. **Erythema.**—This, it is to be remembered, is a
hyperæmic affection, generally transient ; the thickening,
papulation, crusting, scaling, itching, and infiltration of
eczema are never seen in it.

  7. **Favus.**—Where the characteristic yellow, cup-
shaped crusts are present, this disease should never be
mistaken for eczema ; but in a half cured, scaly state I
have seen the scalp with its reddened surface much resemble a squamous eczema capitis. Generally if this

stage has been reached there will already be some of the cicatrices devoid of hair, characteristic of old favus, or if there is any doubt, the withdrawal of all local applications for a week or so would allow a favus to develop its cups, recognizable by the eye ; or, the abundant presence of the parasite could be discovered microscopically, either in the cups if present, or even in the scales and hairs.

8. **Herpes.**—Imperfectly developed patches of zoster or of febrile herpes sometimes resemble eczema considerably, but a well marked case of zoster following a nerve tract should never be mistaken for it. The vesicles of herpes are much more flat than are those of eczema, and are usually grouped together quite differently from the irregular manner in which the lesions of eczema usually appear, and the parts are more painful, even acutely sensitive ; the vesicles of herpes are more persistent than those of eczema, and often dry down without rupturing.

9. **Hydroa.**—The vesicles of hydroa are also generally much larger and more flat than those of eczema, the eruption is apt to be more general than eczema, and there is pain rather than itching.

10. **Impetigo** and Impetigo contagiosa.—Many of the cases formerly called impetigo are now described as pustular eczema, but true impetigo is still recognized by many dermatologists. It consists of separate pustules, superficial in character, with a tendency to scab over and heal, if undisturbed, but with also a tendency to develop new spots elsewhere. In pustular or impetiginous eczema the diseased surface tends to extend until large surfaces may be included in the raw, pus-secreting, scab-covered patches. In impetigo contagiosa the pustules are very superficial, with papery crusts, tending to run together, like pustular eczema ; but there is always a history of contagion, and in the affected person (generally a child) the disease appears to be spread by contact with the secreted matter, new

spots appearing continually, often extending downward from the face; the fingers also very commonly exhibit some or many of the flat, superficial pustules, especially near their extremities.

11. Intertrigo.—It is not always easy or even possible to tell just where intertrigo, or more properly erythema intertrigo, or chafing, ceases and eczema begins. In infants and fat persons we very frequently see quite large, and apparently raw, red surfaces between folds of the skin, as at the nates, beneath the mammæ, etc., which at first sight resemble a moist, red eczema of these regions. But the trouble is a very local one, dependent upon local irritation, as confined sweat and friction, and if properly cared for will pass away almost as suddenly as it appeared. It is simply a hyperæmic condition, due to maceration of the parts with an acrid perspiration; the moisture found on the surface is not thick and sticky as in eczema, but consists of epidermal scales macerated by the perspiration. This condition may, however, run into an eczema in one predisposed thereto, and this state of intertrigo may afford the nidus in which vegetable spores may lodge, producing the so-called eczema marginatum or ringworm of these regions.

12. Lichen.—Lichen simplex and papular eczema are often so nearly alike as almost to defy differentiation in some cases; in general, the papules of lichen tend to occupy the extensor surfaces, those of eczema the flexors; lichen papules are generally grouped, those of eczema are indiscriminately scattered; lichen remains dry and plastic throughout, eczema exudes or presents thickened skin at some time during its course. Lichen planus should always be readily distinguished from eczema by the flat character of the pink, shining papules, with their slightly depressed centres, while the papules of eczema are pointed and bright red. The elements of lichen

planus may become grouped together in large patches, but generally the separate papules can still be distinguished and there are always some new, isolated ones which suffice for a diagnosis. The papules of lichen planus remain papules during their entire course, and leave stains as they disappear; those of eczema often run into other lesions, are of much shorter duration, and do not generally leave discoloration. Both lichen and eczema itch.

13. **Lupus.**—There is little reason for this disease being ever mistaken for eczema, but it is mentioned here because I have seen this happen on a number of occasions. When lupus vulgaris has traversed a large surface, and the skin is red and scaly, eczema might be suspected; but in such a case the separate, soft, pulpy tubercles, which will be found on the edge of the disease establish its character. Lupus erythematosus, if it has considerable of the congestive element and little of the sebaceous, with a red surface and moderate scaling, looks somewhat like erythematous eczema. But here the history, the presence of the sebaceous plugs, and the absence of itching would exclude eczema.

14. **Pemphigus.**—The large bullæ belonging to pemphigus are never seen in eczema, though when the latter are ruptured the crust formed may resemble that of impetiginous eczema. Pemphigus foliaceus is characterized by large flaky exfoliations of epidermis and a raw, tender surface, which, however, does not exude as does an eczematous patch; there is no itching and no thickening.

15. **Pityriasis capitis.** —The scaly pityriasis of the scalp resembles much the chronic scaly eczema; but in the former the scales are more branny, and are moreover heaped up or collected together in considerable thickness, and there may be seen small epidermal prolongations or small epithelial sheaths, from the scales on and around the hairs.

16. **Pityriasis** rubra or **Dermatitis exfoliativa.**—This is distinguished from eczema by the intensity of the redness and the great abundance of the thin, papery scales, and the absence of moisture and thickening   There is some itching, but mainly a burning heat in the skin.   It is a very rare disease.

17. **Phthiriasis.**—Lice in the head give rise to lesions which often resemble pustular eczema very closely; the presence of pediculi and their nits is, however, sufficient for the diagnosis.   But it must also be borne in mind that an eczema of the scalp may by its presence attract pediculi, which then become a secondary element in the case.   In these instances eczema will generally be found elsewhere as well, or the eruption will extend beyond the hairy scalp on to the bare portions of the face, or neck, or ears.   Phthiriasis corporis is sometimes attended with excoriations which might be mistaken for eczema by those unacquainted with the lesions thus produced; the tendency of the insects to locate in the folds of the clothing over the shoulders and about the loins, where their nits may be found adhering to the clothes, furnishes an important diagnostic mark, as most of the lesions are consequently found in these regions.   Crabs, phthiriasis pubis, may give rise to itching and eruptions about the genital region which can be mistaken for eczema.   It is always safe to look first for these parasites and exclude them in cases of eruption in this region.

18. **Prurigo.**—True prurigo, that is, shotty papules, pale red or of the color of normal skin, unless scratched, occurring principally on the legs, attended with great itching and the subsequent development of more or less enlargement of the inguinal glands, is a very rare affection in this country, and need hardly be confounded with eczema.   If the term prurigo is used in the sense in which it is employed in England, the differentiation be-

tween it and papular eczema is indeed difficult. But the tendency to exude in eczema, even in the papular form, the predilection of the eruption for the flexor surfaces in place of the extensors, as in prurigo, and the sharp, inflammatory character, and irregular distribution of the papules of eczema are sufficient to characterize it.

19. **Pruritus.**—Many cases of eczema of the anus and genitals are called "prurigo" or pruritus of these parts, these terms being used indifferently and synonymously by many physicians. There is no such thing as prurigo in this location, and care should be taken to determine whether the trouble is simply one of pruritus or itching, or whether the itching is not a symptom of an eczema; for in the former case applications might be made with the intention of allaying the itching which would do great violence to an eczema. One should also exclude the possibility of the itching being due to the presence of intestinal worms. In pruritus there should be no papules or vesicles, no red, or raw surface, and no thickening of the skin. If there are any cutaneous lesions they will be such only as are caused by the scratching, namely, torn or abraded surfaces. The probabilities in the case of severe and prolonged itching of these parts are greatly in favor of eczema.

With the advent of cold weather we have also a pruritus more or less general, which may be accompanied by marks of much scratching; this has received the name of pruritus hiemalis. The absence of the signs of eczema together with the paroxysmal character of the itching, chiefly about the back, outside of the thighs, calves, and arms, especially on undressing at night, are sufficient to distinguish this from eczema.

20. **Psoriasis.**—A well marked case of psoriasis, with its separate, round, slightly raised, red patches, covered with silvery scales, easily scraped off, together with

the delicate pellicle beneath them, and the bleeding corium under this, need never be confounded with eczema.
When, however, the silvery scales have fallen or have
been removed by treatment, and a red surface is presented, especially if the eruption has run together, forming patches of some size, or if, as frequently occurs on the
legs, the scales are thicker, darker, and more adherent,
the eruption may resemble eczema in a measure.

But respect should be had to the history, which makes
psoriasis always a dry disease, with an uniform eruption;
eczema is polymorphous. Eczema attacks the flexor surfaces by preference, psoriasis the extensors; eczema itches,
psoriasis seldom gives much distress in this way. Psoriasis
of the scalp may be distinguished from eczema by the
greater dryness of the scales, and by the separate, well-
defined patches with healthy tissue between them. The
patches of psoriasis everywhere are sharply outlined, with
rather a tendency to clear in the centre; those of eczema
shade off gradually into healthy skin, and tend to disappear from the margin, and never clear first in the centre.

21. Purpura.—In purpura the eruption being an hem-
orrhagic one, does not fade under pressure; eczema
always pales to a greater or less degree when the finger
is pressed upon it and quickly withdrawn. Sometimes in
an acute attack of purpura the eruption will appear suddenly and be a little elevated, and with a congestive element, and have some burning pain, perhaps a little itching, suggesting eczema; but the differential characters
given should suffice for a diagnosis, when compared with
the features belonging to eczema.

22. Scabies.—Of all diseases psoriasis and scabies are
perhaps the most apt to be mistaken for eczema. The
lesions of scabies are multiform like eczema; papules, vesicles, pustules, and crusts, indeed all the results of inflammation may be present, together with itching. But scabies

has a lesion which eczema cannot have, namely, the little black cuniculi, or burrows of the insect, looking like a bit of dark sewing silk run beneath the skin, and when this can be found with certainty, or an acarus seen microscopically, there is no difficulty in diagnosis. Frequently, however, these furrows have been destroyed by treatment or by scratching, and then as always, we have valuable indications in the history of contagion, which can generally be made out in scabies. Another point of importance is the locality or localities affected. Scabies most commonly appears first on the hands, and especially in the spaces between the fingers, also upon the wrists; likewise about the ankles and soft part of the soles of the feet in children. The penis and scrotum are also very favorite places, and an itchy eruption about the abdomen, with several inflamed points on the penis or scrotum, is strong evidence of scabies. The nipple is also a common place of attack, and itching of the breast without fissured nipples or moist eczematous patches always suggests scabies. The forearms, front edge of the axillæ, and buttocks are also common places for the papules accompanying scabies.

The itching of scabies is much less than that of eczema, it is far more bearable; the former is often spoken of as not unpleasant if scratching is indulged in, whereas the itching of eczema is torture.

But sometimes the diagnosis is exceedingly difficult, for eczema also attacks just the places liable to be affected by scabies, and the diagnosis can be made only by a most careful study of all the features of the case in a totality, and sometimes only by the results of treatment. It is well to remember that scabies does not present the separate patches of eruption seen in eczema, often of some size, and that there is not infiltration of the skin. Sometimes when cases of scabies have been long treated, an artificial eruption is produced by the remedies employed and **we have** lesions resembling papular eczema, perhaps **greatly diffused** over the body.   A suspension of the **irritating** agents, with a little soothing treatment will **generally** soon establish the diagnosis.

23. **Scarlatina.**—Very suddenly developing, finely papular or erythematous eczema, general in distribution or located on the face or neck, might be confounded with the rash of scarlatina, but the general and throat symptoms of the latter should entirely differentiate them.

24. **Small pox.**—Cases are repeatedly suspected to be small pox which are not, and again occasionally the eruption of small pox is supposed to be that of some other affection.   Eczema is perhaps not as likely to be thus confounded as some other eruptions, but an acutely developing eczema, with large papules, on the face and upper part of the body, may resemble small pox in its papular stage.   The general symptoms and the eruption on the hard and soft palate should be sufficient to distinguish the latter, though these may be so slightly marked as to leave room for doubt.   As diagnostic points we have the grouping of the lesions of small pox, the vesiculation on the third day, with umbilication on the fourth or fifth, and pustulation by the sixth day; eczema papules are smaller and irregularly distributed, if vesiculation occurs all are not uniformly affected as in small pox, nor is there umbilication.   There may sometimes be very considerable itching in small pox.

25. **Sycosis.**—The diagnosis between pustular eczema of the bearded face, and true or non-parasitic sycosis, is sometimes most difficult.   But the latter being a perifolliculitis, originating around the deepest part of the root of the hair, it follows that when the pus has travelled along the root and has formed a pustule it has already separated the hair from its attachments, and the hair may

be drawn out without pain. The pustule of eczema, which may also be penetrated by a hair, originates superficially in the papillary layer, and need not have loosened the hair in forming a pustule; hence the hair is extracted from a pustule of eczema of the beard only with great pain. This is true in by far the largest number, but is not necessarily the fact in regard to every pustule; for, in an old standing case of eczema of the beard, the entire thickness of the skin may be so affected, or the hair may have remained in the pustule so long, that the pus has worked down and loosened the hair completely. But, again, eczema is characterized by an erythematous redness between the points, and many papules may be found as well as pustules, and the margin or edge of the eczematous patch fades off insensibly into the healthy skin, as was mentioned in speaking of its differentiation from psoriasis. Moreover, an eczematous patch will often extend out on to parts devoid of hair, whereas, true folliculitis barbæ or sycosis, is by its nature limited to parts bearing large hairs. In sycosis also, we have much deep stinging or pain, in place of the itching of eczema; and further, closely connected with this and dependent likewise upon its pathology, we have a deep seated tenderness in sycosis, when the hairs are seized and pressed downwards into the skin. The diagnosis of eczema from parasitic sycosis, or tinea trichophytina barbæ, will be spoken of shortly, in connection with the diagnosis of ringworm of the rest of the body; also more particularly in connection with eczema of the face.

26. **Syphilis.**—There are not many lesions of syphilis which should be mistaken for eczema, although I remember having seen very many of them thus confounded. It would be impossible here to so describe the differential points which mark all the syphilitic eruptions as to render mistakes impossible, but if due regard be paid to

the symptoms and clinical history of eczema, there should not be much difficulty; the discharge feature and the infiltration of the skin, characteristic of eczema, are wanting in syphilis, nor is there often much if any itching in this latter.

The lesion which may most often be mistaken for eczema is a vesiculo-pustular syphiloderm upon the scalp, to which some have wrongly given the name syphilitic eczema. It is hardly necessary to say that syphilis can never cause true eczema, though eczema may occur on a syphilitic person; but this does not make it a syphilitic eczema. This scalp eruption of syphilis which most resembles eczema is usually composed of small, raw patches, with moderately adherent crusts, either on them or already torn off and adherent to the hairs. Close examination will show that the lesions are really pustular and generally ulcerating, and frequently some of them will have already partially or wholly healed, leaving a cicatrix, which does not occur in eczema.

Syphilis of the palms and soles may sometimes resemble eczema very closely. In the syphilitic eruption, however, careful study will discover that the patches of hardened, scaly eruption are composed of a number of points, papules or tubercles, almost always arranged in circular form, composing the larger patch; the margin will couse quently be irregular or wavy; and it will be somewhat elevated because of the papules or tubercles which compose it. Finally, this edge does not extend by a gradual creeping of the eruption, as eczema spreads insensibly, but by the formation of new, distinct papules at the border of the original patch. This eruption of syphilis may be attended with deep fissures like those in eczema, and there may also often be considerable itching.

Eczematous ulceration of the leg may be mistaken for syphilis, but in my experience the reverse is generally true, namely, that an ulcerating syphilitic eruption is more often called eczema. In long standing eczema of the leg we may have very considerable staining, both in connection with and following the eruption, quite like the conventional "coppery" color so often looked for in syphilis; this is due to the long continued congestion of the capillaries. First it is to be remembered that the ulcerations attending eczema of the leg are more commonly on the lower third, or at least below the middle line, whereas those of syphilis are far more apt to be on the upper portion, or to extend at least above the median line. The ulcerations of eczema of the legs are usually very painful. Syphilitic ulcerations of the leg may or may not be painful; if there is much pain it is apt to take on a nocturnal character, and patients complain rather of a deep boring pain; in ulcerations accompanying eczema they more often describe the sensations to be as though the leg or part would burst, and there is an aching, tired feeling. This latter is due id part to the varicose veins which may often be discovered. Eczematous ulcerations are highly inflammatory in character, the base is apt to be very red and the edges rather everted and hard; if long standing they are generally larger in size than those of syphilis and fewer in number, although syphilitic ulceration may sometimes attain great size. The ulcerations due to syphilis commonly partake of the well-known feature of being composed of a number of smaller lesions compacted together, often with a tendency to circular disposition; the individual points are generally round, the edges of the ulceration are sharply cut, often undermined, and the base indolent, features resulting from the nature of the lesions, namely, an ulceration of previously formed new deposit. The odor from syphilitic ulceration of the leg is usually most fetid, always suggestive of gangrene. Eczema is far more apt to be symmetrical, both legs being affected, whereas the late syphilitic manifestations are commonly one-sided.

Infantile syphilis will sometimes present lesions resembling eczema, especially about the mouth and genital region. Around the mouth we sometimes have a dry, parched condition, slightly scaly and of a brawny red, which may become moist accidentally and look like an erythematous eczema. But close inspection will show that this is composed of separate, large, flat papules, or groups of papules run together in circular form, and presenting characters quite different from the red, moist, or crusting, itchy eczema which belongs to infants: eczema is very rarely confined to the region of the mouth in infants. Sometimes about the anal and genital region we have extensive, red, raw surfaces, which are in fact a combination of the lesions of syphilis and intertrigo, from irritation of some sort. But here we can generally detect the separate lesions of syphilis as described around the mouth, although sometimes the diagnosis must rest on other elements than the features of the eruption alone.

Seldom will one have any of the lesions of syphilis here described as resembling eczema without having at the same time other evidences of the disease which confirm the diagnosis. I do not allude to statements of the patient in reference to previous venereal sores, for this is generally of very little value in establishing the nature of the eruption. But commonly other indications of the disease will be present, or scars of the same, or such clear and definite statements of the existence of lesions as are conclusive

27. Tinea trichophytina.—Ringworm in its different aspects is very frequently confounded with eczema. Upon the scalp, tinea trichophytina capitis, or tinea tonsurans is distinguished from eczema by its circular patches of a dead color, covered with dirty grayish scales, and gen-

erally with a number of broken off hairs. In long standing cases of ringworm of the scalp, the distinct character of the individual patches is lost, and the whole surface may be covered with a grayish scaling, with occasional broken hairs. Eczema in the scalp is very commonly moist at some period, or if of a dry form, it is not in the well-defined circular patches, and the hairs are not broken off, although they may be more or less absent. Where there is a general scaly eczema the scales are of a lighter color, the surface beneath is red, and the eruption very itchy ; ringworm itches little if at all. If there is any doubt in regard to the diagnosis, the surface should be scraped with a dull knife and the debris placed on a slide with a drop of glycerine and liquor potassæ, and examined microscopically. If the disease be parasitic, there will be found parts of the broken hairs, split up at their ends, and they and the scales will be loaded with the sporules of the trichophyton tonsurans.

Ringworm of the body is generally quite easily distinguished from eczema by its red, circular patches, increasing from a small point, and with a tendency to clear in the centre. But occasionally a squamous eczema will appear in separate patches, and may resemble the tinea circinata so closely that much care is necessary to establish the diagnosis with certainty. But in these cases of eczema the spots will appear with almost perfect symmetry on each side of the body, they will not be circular but irregular in outline, and their margins, instead of being sharply defined, as in ring-worm, will fade insensibly into the healthy skin, and they will have no tendency to clear in the centre ; this eczema itches more or less, the ringworm hardly any. Finally, the fungus, which can be detected in the scales scraped from the tinea, is not found on those from the eczema patches.

Ringworm of the beard, tinea barbæ the wrongly

called parasitic sycosis, will always give the history of
spreading from a small point, as in the preceding form, and
often the red, slightly raised, and scaly border of the extending ring can be discovered ; the hairs are lustreless and
often broken off.   Eczema of this region shows the illy-
defined margin common to it, greater uniform redness, and
great itching and burning, and does not give the history of
slow increase from a small point, and does not clear in the
centre.   When an old tinea barbæ has become inflamed,
there are large masses of boggy tissue, elevated, and with
hairs which are dry and dead, standing loose in their follicles ; pustular eczema of the beard does not give these
boggy masses, but is an inflammatory and painful affection
with small pustules, and often a number of crusts ; there is
also generally erythematous eczema adjoining ; whereas in
an inflamed ringworm of the beard, some of the ringed,
superficial disease can generally be discovered.

The so-called eczema marginatum, which is really a
ringworm of the genital and other moist regions, tinea
trichophytina cruris, requires very careful differentiation
from eczema of these parts, because on a perfect recognition of the nature of the eruption will depend the success
of treatment.   Both affections present a raw, red surface,
exceedingly itchy and with a tendency to spread centrifu-
gally.   But in eczema marginatum careful examination will
always demonstrate the presence of an advancing line at
or near the margin of the eruption, which is more red than
the adjoining surface, slightly elevated, and of a height
quite sufficient to be appreciated by the eye.   Together
with this we have a tendency to clear or heal in the centre,
or portion previously occupied, which is characteristic of
all forms of ringworm, the surface left being of a brownish
color, frequently with the new development of small points
of disease, which may again enlarge and travel over the
previously affected area.   This parasitic eruption is gen-

erally engrafted on an eczematous base, or occurs in an eczematous subject, so that the diagnosis may be exceed ingly difficult. Sometimes also the eczema element so predominates that the eruption is to all intents and purposes an eczema, and only after the violence of the inflammation has been subdued can the parasitic element be determined with certainty. Careful microscopic examination will generally reveal the parasite in the debris scraped from the parasitic eruption, though often it is difficult to find.

28. **Urticaria.**—The sudden development of the flat, slightly elevated wheals of urticaria, their rapid disappearance, and the total absence of any moisture or infiltration, even when scratched, should easily exclude any ordinary cases of this eruption. But there is a variety seen, especially in children, namely, urticaria papulosa, known also as lichen urticatus, which often looks very much like a papular eczema. This exhibits scratched papules which often remain some time after the subsidence of the wheal, and appear to constitute the main eruption. But a history of suddenly developing blotches will always be given, and generally a slight erythematous halo left by the wheal may be seen around most of the papules. It is not very uncommon for urticaria to develop with or subsequent to eczema ; remembering well the characteristics of the two, they should be easily differentiated.

We have thus seen that this polymorphous eruption eczema may at times resemble most of the eruptions which are common, and some which are rare, and that there is no one single, distinct, and pathognomonic sign or symptom by means of which it can always be immediately diagnosticated. But we have also seen that there are features which characterize each and every eruption with which eczema could be confounded, which, if they are all well and carefully attended to, will render the differences clear. It will therefore be appreciated that the remark made at the opening of the chapter was not without foundation, namely, that eczema in many cases must be recognized not only by its own proper symptoms, but also by the exclusion of the other affections which the particular case may resemble.

It will be noticed that little mention has been made of the vesicle in eczema. Older writers classed eczema as a vesicular eruption, and this feature has become so impressed upon the general professional mind that one constantly sees physicians searching for vesicles as an evidence of the eczematous nature of an eruption. This view of the essential character of the eruption of eczema has been and will be the cause of innumerable mistakes of diagnosis if persisted in, for it will abundantly appear from what has been said in this chapter and in other chapters that very many cases never present a vesicle from their beginning to their termination; if vesicles do appear they are generally very short lived. Among a hundred miscellaneous cases of acute and chronic eczema, as they are first presented for treatment, it may be safely asserted that not ten cases, if indeed five, would present a single well-marked vesicle.

PROGNOSIS.

The prognosis of eczema depends upon so many different elements, that it is difficult to speak at once positively in regard to any particular case. It may be stated however, unreservedly, that eczema is a curable disease, and that proper care and knowledge on the part of the physician and patient, can succeed in entirely curing it.

The expression "curable disease" is used intelligently and intentionally, for there is little or no tendency in eczema to a spontaneous cure; its natural course is to persist indefinitely, and even to defy treatment in many cases.

But there are few diseases which demonstrate, on the

other hand, the controlling power of rightly directed management more perfectly or satisfactorily, and in a manner about which there can be no doubt, than this same eczema. An eruption which has made itself painfully manifest for months or years, is arrested by the measures advised, and after a period ceases to exist; there can be no doubt whatever, about cause and effect in such a case.

While, however, as a disease eczema can be successfully managed, individual cases may and constantly do give much trouble; so many elements are concerned in the cure of eczema, the habits, constitution, diet, mode of life, occupation, antecedents, etc., that, as before stated, the prognosis in regard to individual cases must often be guarded. If the right measures are employed, according to our present light, the disease can be and is removed as a rule, although often it is a matter of months or years.

It will be understood that in these remarks upon prognosis, reference is not made simply to removing the local eruption present, which indeed may sometimes prove a troublesome task, but also relates to breaking up the state or disposition underlying this, so that when the local lesion is removed the skin remains free.

But, undoubtedly, many cases are not cured even when exactly the right management is directed, because it so often happens that for some reason or other the precise rules are not, or cannot be executed to a letter. For the successful management of the disease every detail, both those relating to local treatment, and also to hygienic, dietetic, and constitutional measures, must be minutely carried out, and often for some considerable time even after the skin lesion has disappeared.

It will be seen therefore that the prognosis depends very greatly upon the treatment, and this again often far more upon the patient than upon the physician. The cure of obstinate eczema may sometimes involve a very radical change in the life and surroundings of the individual, and his occupation ; it may involve change of climate and visits to mineral springs, etc.   Finally, the prognosis of eczema may depend upon results of treatment of other organs, as when the disease is dependent upon ovarian or uterine disorder, or when rebellious dyspepsia keeps up an eczema of the hands or face, or profound nervous depression is the underlying cause.

To give a prognosis in eczema, therefore, the patient requires to be studied and understood, and, as will be judged, may require very varied treatment : treated empirically with arsenic and oxide of zinc ointment alone, the prognosis of eczema must generally be bad.

Certain forms of eczema, however, differ very greatly in regard to their course and tendencies.   Acute vesicular eczema generally yields readily, whereas the papular and erythematous forms are more rebellious : recurrences are always to be judged cautiously.   When infiltration exists to any great extent, its removal is often a matter of weeks or months.

The locality affected often influences the prognosis considerably.   Eczema of the palms is exceedingly rebellious, as also some cases of erythematous eczema about the mouth ; separate patches on the extremities or trunk, also upon the face of children yield much more readily. The prognosis of the eruption as it affects different localities will be mentioned later on.   The eruption cannot be driven from one locality to another, although if it is treated by external measures alone while the internal causes remain, other patches of disease are very likely to appear upon various localities.

In regard to the fear often expressed that some danger or harm may come from curing a long-standing eczema, it may be definitely stated that there is absolutely no foundation for this whatever.   Rightly managed, only *good* can result to the patient from the line of treatment most suitable for the eczema: one constantly hears the statement that the patient feels and appears much better in general health than for a long period previous to undergoing treatment. Nor is there even any danger in rightly treating the eruption locally; in Vienna the plan of local treatment is almost exclusively employed, and those who write and teach there, as well as those who follow the clinics, all testify that no harm ever results therefrom.

Although exceedingly rarely if ever fatal, eczema, by the long continued irritation arising therefrom, may exhaust greatly the patient's health and strength, and intercurrent diseases may then destroy life. But, as demonstrated elsewhere, this event certainly is not to be regarded as a "striking in" of the eruption, such an occurrence is unknown to scientific or practical medicine. The cure of the disease in the most rapid and best manner affords the surest and quickest prospects of restoration to perfect health and strength of one afflicted with eczema.

CHAPTER VI.

NATURE OF ECZEMA.—CONSTITUTIONAL OR LOCAL.

THE suggestion of a local pathology of diseases of the skin is of comparatively recent date, and stands in bold contrast to the older humoralistic doctrine, which ascribed all these diseases to a morbid entity, a *materies morbi,* which seeks exit from the system through the skin, and whose escape is beneficial ; and the positive demonstration within the present century of a local cause of several cutaneous maladies (such as dermatitis, the parasitic affections, etc.) which had, for ages, been regarded as expressions of blood states, is an achievement of which modern dermatology may justly be proud.

This discovery of a local origin of certain skin lesions, and the fact of the resemblance between some of the forms of artificial eruptions and the lesions of impetigo, lichen, eczema, etc., have led some to claim, still further, that most, if not all, of the diseases affecting the skin are either the results of local external causes, or are local diseases originating in idiopathically deranged action of the elements of the skin. The adoption of this view has undoubtedly been promoted by a natural reaction from the too exclusively humoral doctrines previously entertained.

It need hardly be said that in arguing a constitutional origin and nature of eczema, I do not desire at all to return to the older humoralistic doctrine of disease, but shall seek to keep entirely within the bounds of recent chemical physiology and pathology. Nor is it desired to ignore the importance of local cell-action, for, most certainly the great organ of the skin is capable of taking on diseased action from cold and various agencies, quite as much as any other organ of the body ; the elements composing it may undergo inflammation, hypertrophy, atrophy, or perverted development and growth. But, as will appear later, a local pathology fails to account for all the phenomena presented in eczema, while general and constitutional conditions, and the results of therapeutics afford incontrovertible indications of internal causation and relations.

The local pathology of eczema has rested largely on three grounds : first, on the results obtained in the local treatment of this and other diseases of the skin, especially in the larger hospitals in Europe, notably that in Vienna ; second, upon microscopical researches in histology ; and, third, on a clinical and microscopic study of the artificial eruptions produced on the skin by irritating substances, idiopathically and experimentally. First a word in regard to the last of these, and then they will all be considered at length in connection with other matters.

Now, while there is as yet no absolute proof that the pathological process excited artificially in the skin differs essentially from that taking place in acute eczema, we need not conclude that eczema is of local origin because its eruption resembles artificial dermatitis. If we accept one artificial eruption as eczema, we must accept all as such, from the large blisters following cantharides, heat, and cold, to the discrete, pustular eruption produced by croton oil or tartar emetic, or the slight erythematous blush caused by the mildest irritant. Moreover, many of these artificial eruptions resemble erysipelas even more than they do eczema, and yet there will be few who will hold that true erysipelas is a local disease of the skin ; again, the eruptions of croton oil and tartar emetic resemble those of smallpox and syphilis, without this being an argument against the constitutional nature of these latter ; while the eruptions produced by the insect in scabies and by lice are frequently confounded with eczema. These lesions are all purely local, there is simply a local response of the cells and capillaries of the over-stimulated part ; they are all but forms and varieties of inflammation of the skin, and are properly termed dermatitis, and bear no more relation to eczema than does the inflammation of a sprained joint to true rheumatism. In a very small proportion of persons, such irritations may become the starting point of true eczema, but in them I believe that the elements of the ecze-matous diathesis may always be discovered. A demon-stration of the essential difference between these artificial eruptions and eczema is shown by the fact that it is not uncommon to induce dermatitis, by a blister or by caustic potash, for the cure of chronic eczema.

It is necessary, therefore, in the present study to remember the distinction between eczema and dermatitis, for undoubtedly much that is often treated for the former is but the latter, and of course no argument can be drawn from therapeutical results obtained in dermatitis as to the local nature of eczema.

Before proceeding systematically to examine the several points regarding the local or constitutional nature of ec-zema, let us consider, for a moment, the question of the possibility of a double origin, whether it can own two na-tures, being sometimes local and sometimes constitutional. In regard to the skin lesions in the contagious exanthe-mata and syphilis, no question exists that their origin is solely and always due to the introduction of a poison, which acts through the system, and that the cutaneous manifesta-tions are but one exhibition of their effect. Passing now to such general diseases as gout and rheumatism, whose etiology is more deeply hidden, we do not doubt that the local phenomena observed in each are always the result of the same constitutional condition; some of the earlier links in the chain of cause and effect are recognized in the functional derangement of certain organs, and a consequent sub-oxidation or imperfect elaboration of the elements of food, and an absence of healthy disintegration of tissue. When, therefore, we speak of cold or external injury as being the cause of gouty or rheumatic inflammatory action in a part, we understand readily that it is only intended to signify that it was the *exciting cause*, which determined that that particular spot should be affected, or that the disease should develop at that particular time. The same line of thought might be extended to other diseases, showing that it is irrational to deny the constitutional origin of a disease unless its local nature can be established in a manner answering every requirement, as is the case in the parasitic diseases of the skin ; quite as impossible is it to exclude a local exciting causation in addition, when the constitutional nature fails to account for every condition.

Great error has, therefore, been made, I believe, by those who look only or mainly at the local causes, and argue therefrom a local nature of eczema, they forgetting the established principles in general medicine in regard to *predisposing* and *exciting* causes of disease. This is verified by the fact of the impossibility of producing chronic eczema artificially, at will, in a person not subject thereto either in self or family.

Our conclusions then, thus far, are that eczema cannot be both a local and a constitutional disease, that is, either exclusively, according to the case ; and that the eruptions resembling eczema, artificially produced, are either ordinary dermatitis, with a strong tendency to spontaneous recovery, or are true eczema in eczematous subjects, in whom the exciting cause, instead of occurring in the ordinary way, has been artificially supplied, just as a gouty person might, by measures voluntarily applied, induce a true gouty inflammation of a joint.

In the further study of the question as to whether eczema is a local disease of the skin or a manifestation of constitutional disorder, I propose to develop the following points :

(1) The nature and character of the eruption in disorders of the skin which are recognized to be constitutional, as the contagious fevers, syphilis, etc., drawing a comparison between eczema and these affections, and showing their points of resemblance.

(2) The nature and character of local diseases of the skin.

(3) The microscopic anatomy of eczema, with a view to its comparison with that of the local skin diseases on the one hand, and with that of the constitutional on the other.

(4) The clinical history of eczema, in so far as it bears on the question ; the points considered being (*a*) age, (*b*) sex, (*c*) location of eruption, (*d*) relapses, (*e*) hereditary transmission, (*f*) gouty and strumous symptoms, (*g*) urinary disturbances, (*h*) bronchitis, etc.

(5) The clinical history of some local diseases, to show the differentiating elements between constitutional disorders and those believed to be local, as epithelioma, verruca, keloid, parasitic and mechanical diseases of the skin, etc.

(6) The effect of local treatment, and how far the success of local measures necessitates a belief in the purely local nature of the disease.

(7) The effect of constitutional treatment, and the internal and general measures of service in eczema, to show how far their effect proves that the disease which they remove is constitutional.

(1) In comparing eczema to the acknowledged constitutional disorders affecting the skin, contagious fevers, leprosy, syphilis, etc., we must not, of course, press the similar-

ity too far. We find, however, certain resemblances, as in the symmetry of development of the lesions, for eczema, if uninfluenced by local causes, will, when carefully studied, be found to exhibit this very strikingly ; the peripheral mode of spreading of eczema resembles much that of erysipelas, and the scattered eruption sometimes seen corresponds much to the mode of development of other exanthematous diseases, including syphilis. Eczema also is not infrequently attended with fever in its more acute and general forms. The characters of the lesions in eczema are not entirely unlike those of constitutional diseases, which are marked by, first, congestion ; second, peri-vascular exudation ; and, third, if these former have been sufficiently severe, desquamation. The lesions of eczema are also superficial, and rarely, if ever, do they leave cicatrices, when uncomplicated.

(2) In contrast with these stand the characteristics of local diseases of the skin, marked by their utter want of symmetry (unless accidental), their extension depending either on a recognized cause, or being unexplainable, as in keloid, epithelioma, etc. ; local diseases very rarely affect the whole integument, or even large portions, unless ichthyosis, of whose true nature, however, we know very little, be granted as such. Local diseases, moreover, acknowledge no constitutional connections nor fever ; while, finally, the congestive element of eczema stands in striking contrast to its absence in local diseases, except, of course where it is called forth by local stimulation. I am well aware that certain cases of eczema present some of the features of local disease ; but this is the exception, whereas it is rare to find exceptions in regard to local diseases exhibiting any constitutional features ; and, as we have concluded that eczema cannot be at one time a local and at another a constitutional disease, the weight of evidence is decidedly in favor of the internal origin of eczema.

(3) The study of the microscopic anatomy of eczema throws but little light on its etiology, but the main points in its histology will be seen to favor the constitutional rather than the local nature of this affection. The first anatomical change observable in eczema is capillary congestion, resulting in capillary stasis and exudation in the tissue of the skin, producing more or less œdema. In some instances the process stops here, or is arrested by treatment, and we have only the erythematous state, followed by moderate desquamation, the result of the impaired nutrition of the outer layers of the skin, a state very similar to the epithelial shedding in scarlatina, erysipelas, or measles.

If the exudation is too great to allow of absorption, it seeks egress through the external layers of the skin, or becomes organized as chronic infiltration. When the outer surface is still intact, the hard, horny epidermis resists further progress and a vesicle forms; when the epidermal layer has been dissolved off or ruptured, the fluid oozes from the surface.

In chronic eczema, the exuded plasma has become organized, and is seen as cell infiltration of the corium; the papillæ are much enlarged; the lymphatics, both in the papillæ and corium, are increased in size and dilated; the bloodvessels are sometimes obliterated and even the deepest parts of the skin are involved.

We will now consider for a moment some views in regard to the local nature of eczema propounded by Dr. Tilbury Fox, in the Lettsomian Lectures for 1869 and 1870. He suggests that the capillary congestion is a *consequence* of cell-activity, arguing that mere capillary excitement cannot give rise to eczema, because otherwise the erythemata would constantly overstep their limits. The element of the influence of the nervous system is largely considered by Dr. Fox, who believes that this abnormal state of the cells may be in response to "perverted innervation," as suggested by Hebra some time since ; but while Hebra limited the action of the nerve influence to the production of "congestion and other disturbances of the circulation," Fox considers its influence in inducing cell proliferation a very necessary point to be admitted in eczema.

That independent cell-action has much to do with inflammatory and other changes in the skin, is evident from the results of mechanical and chemical irritation, where, as in the case of the ordinary blister, the intervention of any blood influence cannot be suggested with reason ; but that the cells are under very direct control of the nervous system is also very plain from the lesions in zoster, elephantiasis Græcorum, those occurring after nerve injuries, etc. ; here the cells which under normal nerve control absorb just enough nutriment to maintain their proper relations, under perverted nerve control take on morbid action.

But while a step in advance is made in recognizing the direct agency of the cell elements of the skin in the production of the lesions of eczema (and independent cell activity can be no longer denied, as is shown in leucocytes), and while the influence of the nervous system in the production of cell changes is acknowledged, there is yet no proof that this cell-change is really primary in eczema, and independent of constitutional conditions, and that it exists as a local affair ; and this view finds little support beyond theory. Should, however, repeated, careful, and well verified microscopic studies demonstrate cell change in the earliest erythematous stages of eczema, and possibly also in the skin of eczematous patients before or after disease, it would do much to enlighten what otherwise must remain uncertain, namely, the part that the diseased tissues take in eczema, how far they are primary and how far secondary. For the present, therefore, the constitutional relations of eczema are so abundant and conclusive that they must be granted to be of stronger weight.

(4) We will next turn to a consideration of the constitutional relations of eczema, as exhibited in its clinical history.   In regard to the age at which it occurs, we have
found that eczema affects all, from the cradle to the grave;
none are too young, none too old to suffer from it.   This
is more the character of constitutional than of local disease;
cancerous affections seldom, if ever, are seen in the young;
warts (of the ordinary variety) seldom in the old ; keloid
very generally in middle life, both extremes being spared.
The vegetable parasitic diseases rarely occur in the old ;
whereas again in them are found changes in the skin, and
diseases therefrom, not seen in young life.

Eczema occurs about as frequently in the male as in
the female.   In location, eczema spares no part of the surface, and, I believe, may affect every portion of the mucous
membrane as well, while its development is very commonly
symmetrical ; these features are those of a general and constitutional disease rather than of one of local nature.   The
tendency to recurrence in the same parts might be claimed
as a local feature in eczema ; but here it is often evidently
due to the same exciting cause again and again ; and it
must also be conceded that tissues are undoubtedly weakened by disease, and are therefore more likely to be affected the second time than are sound tissues ; this is observed in gout and rheumatism, as also in affections of the
mucous membranes.

But relapses in eczema furnish further indications of a
constitutional nature, for fresh attacks of eczema are very
commonly found to follow a depression of vitality, and the
eruption by no means occupies the same location each time.
I have frequently observed that the spots of eczema fall
almost if not quite as often on new tissue as on exactly
the sites of a former disease.

If the claim of an inherited, perverted tendency of tissue formation could be established in eczema, which ten-

dency lies dormant until called into activity by some exciting cause, it would still fail to explain alone why a cause
which is at one time inefficacious, will, on another occasion,
even in a much less degree, be sufficient to produce the
disease ; whereas the constitutional relations of eczema
give this explanation.   That patients with eczema are the
frequent subjects of the systemic derangements connected
with or tending toward gout, as well as of the complete
manifestations of this disease, is very certain ; this observation is of ancient date, and is strikingly confirmed by recent
science. It is not very uncommon to find attacks of gout
alternating with those of eczema, and clinical study shows
that various disorders which may properly be classed under
the name of functional derangements of the liver are very
common in the subjects of this disease of the skin.

These systemic disorders are shown in the urine,
which undergoes functional derangement in a large proportion of the cases of eczema.   In a recent contribution to
and study of the subject by the writer,* the following conclusions were reached : "Eczema patients seldom pass
large amounts of urine, the tendency being to scanty secretion, almost always unnaturally acid, with a specific gravity
averaging above normal.   Free uric acid, the urates, and
oxalate of lime abound ; sometimes oxaluria is very persistent.   Albumen is rarely seen.   The urea and uric acid
are often below the normal standard, although they may
be in excess when a large portion of the integument is
affected ; indican has been found in pathological quantities.   When the specific gravity is high, it may be due to
an increase in the sulphates.   The chlorides are diminished."

It may be claimed that these urinary changes are observed in persons also presenting no cutaneous disease,
and that therefore there is no connection between the two.

* Archives of Dermatology, October, 1875. p. 1.

I am not yet in a position to prove exactly what changes in the urine necessarily accompany eczema, but mention those that have been actually observed to show that patients with these diseases are not in the perfect health often claimed for them, and, although a casual examination will often fail to detect any disease other than that of the outer integument, I assert that searching investigation will generally demonstrate elements of disordered health, very commonly shown in the condition of the urine. And as these are removed by appropriate remedies the eczema improves, and *vice versa*.

Not less striking, as indicative of the constitutional relations of eczema, is the occurrence of bronchitis and asthma, conjointly or alternately, in the patient, or in his immediate family; the truth of this is well attested by many writers, and constantly observed by myself.

The neurotic clinical relations of eczema are also very interesting, and indicate other than a local nature of the disease. This subject is more fully developed in another chapter, and need but be mentioned here.

(5) Enough has perhaps already been said in reference to the clinical history of *local diseases* of the skin, but a few points may be again alluded to with advantage in connection with what has just preceded. No constitutional relations have been recognized, to my knowledge, in any of these; constitutional remedies have no effect upon them. Their unsymmetrical character and irregular development have been mentioned, as also their removal solely by local measures. Local diseases of the skin of external origin are represented by the parasitic affections and dermatitis; idiopathic misbehavior of cells is exemplified by epithelioma and keloid; herpes zoster may be taken as a type of an acute local disease of the skin dependent on nerve elements; and ichthyosis perhaps, of a chronic, local disturbance of general cell nutrition; the clinical history

of each of these is familiar to all, and quite different from that of eczema.

Hebra, as is well known, has always stood as the representative of local pathology and therapeutics, and it may not be uninteresting or unprofitable to refer briefly to his latest views in regard to the purely local nature of eczema, as found in the recent second edition of his work.[*] That I may not be charged with misunderstanding him, I will quote a section from the close of the long chapter on the Etiology of Eczema (p. 462). After repeating what had been said in the former edition to show the local nature of the disease, and after stating his disbelief in any diathetic cause, he however says : "While, therefore, we cannot accede to any peculiar herpetic dyscrasia, we must, on the other hand, confirm the fact that certain conditions of the human organism, partly transient, partly permanent, at one time increase and at another time diminish its susceptibility to agencies producing eczema. These physical conditions are called a disposition, or predisposing cause, *momentum disponens*, to distinguish them from the direct exciting cause of irritating agencies, and we are obliged to recognize these elements in the etiology of eczema, because experience confirms it."

"For example, we see an eczema on the hands and forearms of a young girl who has been engaged in washing soiled linen, and we declare that the origin of the eczema is in the action of the lye, soap, hot water, and friction. Now, at the same time with this girl, there are many other females washing the same linen in the same lye, using the same soap, etc., without acquiring eczema. Indeed, this very girl who now has eczema, has for many years been exposed to the same influences without becoming affected. What is the general cause of her present susceptibility? A careful examination of her general condition will give

* Lehrbuch der Hautkrankheiten, Zweite Aufl. ; Erlangen. 1874.

the explanation.   The girl who before was healthy, robust, and regular in her menses, has now lost her appetite, has become sluggish and languid, her appearance is pale and bloated, her menstruation is profuse ; in a word, she has become chlorotic, and thereby eczematous.   The remedies suitable for the chlorosis are now employed ; the appetite and power of work return, the menses become regular, and the eczema disappears in spite of the continued washing and exposure to the influence of the agencies causing it. The same observation is made in reference to pregnant and nursing women ; also in those suffering from chronic sexual disturbances.   The latter must always be looked upon as favoring elements (a *momentum disponens*, or predisposing cause), which induce a *status minoris resistentiæ*, and allow an otherwise ordinary skin irritant to become an exciting cause, a *momentum excitans*."

After again claiming that we need no blood explanation of eczema, Hebra adds : " In order not to be misunderstood, we will, however, here again state that every eczema is not caused by a local irritation, but that it may be occasioned by diseases of the rest of the system."

Such clear and unqualified statements as to the constitutional nature and origin of eczema are unexpected from one so prominently known in connection with local pathology, and show that his opinions had latterly undergone considerable change.   It must be remembered, however, that at the time of the first edition of Hebra's work, in 1860, upon which his reputation as a local pathologist greatly rests, many of the crude theories of the past had not yet been completely overthrown ; and also that within his experience many diseases which had formerly been considered constitutional, had been demonstrated to be purely local, as scabies, the vegetable parasitic diseases, plica polonica, etc., and that the success of local measures in these seemed to demonstrate to him that other affections were also local ; he had, however, the candor to acknowledge his mistake fourteen years later.

(6) We come now to one of the most interesting and at the same time most disputed portions of our investigation, namely, the relative effects of local and constitutional treatment as indicating the nature of eczema. Hebra and Neumann declare, in the most positive terms, that it is quite unnecessary to regard the constitutional relations of this disease, except when they are striking, and those who have followed these teachers for any length of time can testify how completely this idea is carried out in the Vienna General Hospital. External remedies and measures are used there almost exclusively, it being the greatest exception to have any questions asked in regard to the general health ; and internal medication, it may safely be asserted, is very rarely, if ever, employed in the Hospital, in eczema, except by way of experiment ; and yet this eruption is removed in a very satisfactory manner. Does this, however, prove the local nature of the disease ? In answer to this I need but suggest how the stiffness resulting from gouty and rheumatic inflammation is benefited by external counter-irritants and passive motion, while the origin of the serous inflammation and fibrous thickening is recognized as of constitutional origin. Syphilitic iritis may be subdued by atropine alone, and tubercular laryngitis receive great benefit from topical treatment ; the ulcers of dysentery may be cured, and the discharge of leucorrhœa arrested, and yet these diseases be manifestations of constitutional states. In regard to the successful treatment of acute eczema by local measures alone, I need only recall that, as the acute attacks of gout are in a measure self-limited, while the constitutional state remains, so the local manifestations of acute eczema may subside if not aggravated by external circumstances, that is if properly treated and protected, while the constitutional state connected therewith remains.

But there is hardly the slightest influence exerted by local treatment in preventing the return of eczema, whereas we know that constitutional measures have power to prevent relapses. Again, in this country at least, local measures often fail to accomplish the desired end until constitutional measures are resorted to in addition. In considering the effect of local treatment as an argument for the local nature of eczema, it is well to bear in mind the distinction between dermatitis and eczema, for many cases treated as the latter disease are often entirely local in character, the result of local irritants, possessing in themselves a strong tendency to heal when the irritating cause is removed and the inflamed surfaces protected; that is, these are cases of dermatitis and not of eczema.

I believe true eczema to be a constitutional state wherein ordinary irritants give rise to inflammatory changes in the skin, which form an important element of the disease, but which are no more its sole element than the cutaneous phenomena of the exanthemata, leprosy, syphilis, etc., or the joint lesions of gout and rheumatism are the sole manifestations of these maladies. I believe also that single attacks of eczema correspond in nature very much to those of such diseases as gout and rheumatism, in which the local changes have a greater or less tendency to self-limitation, although the effects of the disease may long remain. That is, as arthritic, pulmonary, or cerebral symptoms appear to be the culmination of blood-processes which we know as gout and rheumatism, so eczema is directly dependent upon a somewhat similar, although as yet little defined, blood change, the acute symptoms corresponding to those of rheumatism and gout, while the chronic local alterations in the skin answer to the gouty concretions on and in the synovial membranes, and to the rheumatic thickening of the valves of the heart or around joints long inflamed; and, as in gout and rheumatism, there is a tendency for the attacks to recur again and again, the health in the interval seeming to be perfect, so in eczema the local phenomena may be manifested from time to time, without any very apparent constitutional disorder between. It may also happen that the constitutional state may pass away spontaneously or under dietary, hygienic, and medicinal measures, while the *product* of the disease, the infiltration and consequent itching remain.

Now but little can be done to arrest the acute phenomena of eczema by local means, other than by protective and soothing applications ; but the *results* may be removed by local stimulants, which induce cell activity within the bounds of health. I speak especially of this disease in adults, for infantile eczema exhibits more plainly the constitutional elements, whose great activity often renders local measures very futile.

While, therefore, the arguments are against eczema *being* a local disease of the skin, it must be admitted that it may *become* a local disease in its skin lesions, and as such may be amenable very largely to local treatment, as far as relates to the single manifestations of disease at any one time.

(7) Whatever may be the views of those who hold exclusively to the value of local treatment in eczema, no doubt whatever exists in my own mind, nor, as far as I can learn, in the mind of a large share of those who make skin affections a special study, that constitutional measures are both valuable and necessary to the cure of most cases of this disease. And by constitutional treatment I do not mean arsenic alone, nor any one specific remedy, for truth demands the acknowledgment that specifics for diseases do not exist, unless it be with such exceptions as mercury for syphilis and quinine for malaria. But by constitutional treatment I understand the employment of every measure for the cure of disease which cannot truly be called local treatment.

As has been already stated, it will be found that most patients with eczema present anomalies in their urinary secretion, and in proportion as this exists will the congestive feature of the disease be marked, and in the same proportion will it be seen that the disease is benefited by cathartic and diuretic remedies. A not inconsiderable number of patients with eczema are habitually constipated, and the disease will often resist all local and other measures until this is remedied. Many are what is called bilious, and nitric acid will do more to cure their skin disease than any other means. It is not at all uncommon, in this country, to find eczema in those who are extremely nervous, and cases are constantly met with where an enormous mental strain is keeping up the disease; here the constitutional measure of rest, with perhaps change of scene and climate, is imperatively demanded, together with nerve tonics of various kinds. In dispensary practice in this city a good portion of all eczematous patients exhibit the features known as strumous or scrofulous, and are more quickly and surely cured by the internal administration of cod-liver oil than by any other remedy, local medication either being used not at all, or playing a very unimportant part. Arsenic also is sometimes capable of entirely curing, that is, removing, eczema, and that tolerably quickly, without the use of any local measures whatever, as I have repeatedly witnessed. Iron is indicated in a large share of our eczematous patients; others require such remedies as rhubarb and soda; and the vegetable tonics play an important rôle in our therapeusis. Diet, hygiene, exercise, and bathing, are all essential in my opinion to a successful management of this disease.

The fact that patients who have been thus carefully managed not only recover from the individual attack under proper local measures much more quickly than when the latter alone are used, but that they most certainly are in a better condition to resist future attacks, and that relapses are far less frequent, points strongly toward a constitutional origin of the disease. The action of these measures is not local, is not directed to the skin; but by virtue of the influence exerted on the general economy, as well as on the affected tissues, they cure the disease in question. The argument from this is therefore conclusive of the internal or constitutional nature of eczema.

In this study I have not referred much to the views of writers on dermatology, because, with the exceptions which I have mentioned from time to time, the opinion is very general that eczema is a constitutional disorder. By a constitutional disorder, as we now understand it, is not meant the existence of some peccant material or *materies morbi*, which the system endeavors to throw off; nor that the discharge is in any way curative or beneficial to the system; nor that the removal of the cutaneous lesion can in any way or manner act prejudicially to the economy; but the expression, constitutional disorder, is understood in the same sense in which it can be applied to gout, rheumatism, leucocythæmia, scorbutus, etc. And it is used here in especial distinction from local disease—that is a pure and specific disease of the tissues of the skin itself, singly and alone—as the artificial eruptions, parasitic diseases, epithelioma, verruca, keloid, etc.

Vaccination is another process which we not rarely see followed by eczema; do we suppose here a local cause (other than exciting), that is, does it induce any change in the cells of the skin whereby they are more prone to eczema? I believe not, because of the very general adoption of vaccination, and the very few cases of eczema immediately following; I need hardly state that there can, of course, be no blood-poisoning, no contagion of eczema by means of the lymph, even when taken from

a vaccinifer suffering from eczema ; we know of no transmission by this means except that of syphilis, unless it
be a tendency to carbuncular inflammation, of which I
have observed a number of cases, and which others occasionally meet with.   The only agency which vaccination
can exert in calling forth an eczema, is, I believe, simply
that of a local irritant, acting in the same way as a burn
or other excessive stimulation, to start the eruption in
one predisposed thereto.

Equally useless and uncertain is it, in my judgment,
to look upon dentition in any other light than as an exciting cause, not acting locally, it is true, but probably as
a reflex irritation, and as such I believe it to be of more
or less importance ; but in view of the small proportion
of teething infants who have eczema severely, other
elements must be looked to for the real etiology of this
disease ; this is shown also by the frequent occurrence of
eczema in those of older years, and also before the teeth
begin to appear.

Erroneous diet, however, I consider as an all-important
and undoubtedly prolific cause of eczema in infants, as will
be discussed later : this point is mentioned here only as an
argument in favor of the constitutional origin of the disease
under consideration.

That local causes are of very great importance in the
etiology of eczema in infants, as well as in adults, is beyond doubt ; such causes are the use of irritating diaper-
linen, harsh bandages, too frequent and careless washing
and drying, incautious exposure of the face to cold air, hot
caps on the head, harsh attempts to remove the dried sebaceous matter from the scalp, etc. ; but that the disease
very frequently does not get well upon the removal of
these irritants, and under local measures alone, is certain,
and that a proper study and direction of constitutional
measures will cure the disease, if proper local treatment

is employed, or even without local treatment, is equally sure.

In the succeeding chapter it will be seen that struma, or the scrofulous state is among the predisposing causes of eczema. For the proper study of this relation, we need to have the true position of scrofula more clearly defined than at present, its causes and symptoms more sharply drawn, and further statistical details recorded. That quite a share of children with eczema, among the poor, exhibit some of the features called scrofulous, that is, pale, pasty skins, light hair, eyes, and complexion, enlarged glands, ophthalmia, otorrhœa, etc., is not to be questioned, and that this state has also special effect in causing eczema, by its depressing power, cannot now be doubted. It is certain that eczema exhibits somewhat different features when occurring in these subjects from those shown in patients of a gouty habit; the tendency to pus formation is evident in the secretion from eczema seen in those presenting the phenomena known as strumous.

The results of this inquiry as to the local or constitutional nature of eczema may be summed up in the following propositions :

I. Eczema is a disease *sui generis*, and is not to be confounded in any way with other states; as, with artificial dermatitis, the eruption from lice, scabies, etc.

II. Eczema cannot own a double, independent causation, or nature, at one time local, and at another constitutional ; but, with other diseases, may have a twofold cause, namely, a predisposing internal or general, and an exciting local cause.

III. Eczema in many of its features resembles the accepted constitutional diseases more than it does those recognized as local.

IV. The skin lesions of eczema, as also its micro-scopical characters, more nearly resemble those of the general and constitutional diseases affecting the skin, than those of purely local diseases.

V. Eczema is very properly likened to catarrh of the mucous membranes, but no argument as to its local nature can be drawn therefrom; it is very probable that some proportion of the mucous attacks called catarrh are eczema of this tissue.

VI. Eczema resembles gout and rheumatism, in certain respects, and is dependent upon a somewhat similar, although as yet unknown, constitutional cause; many of the skin lesions, as ordinarily observed, must be looked upon as the *local results* of the disease, removable by local means.

VII. There as yet exists no microscopical or physi-ological proof that eczema is the sole result of local cell disorder, either congenital, acquired, or due alone to per-verted nerve action; although from our present knowl-edge of independent cell activity, and from the intimate connection between nerve elements and the cells com-posing the skin, it is highly probable that cell action and nerve influence are important factors in eczema.

VIII. Local causes may at times play a very im-portant part in determining attacks of eczema, but are in-capable alone of producing the disease. In the larger share of instances no sufficient local cause can be made out.

IX. The clinical history of eczema furnishes much evidence of constitutional relations, mainly with conditions allied to gout, rheumatism and the scrofulous state.

X. Local treatment alone is often insufficient to re-move the lesions of eczema, and cannot prevent or delay relapses; its occasional success does not demonstrate the local nature of this affection.

XI. Constitutional treatment, alone and singly, can cure many cases of eczema and prevent or delay relapses in a certain proportion of cases; by constitutional treatment is intended every agency not properly placed among local measures.

XII. The total weight of evidence and argument is that eczema is a manifestation of constitutional disorder, and not a purely local disease of the skin.

CHAPTER VII.

In the preceding chapter, in which was considered the question as to whether eczema was a local disease of the skin or a manifestation of constitutional disorder, the weight of evidence and argument was found to be conclusively in favor of a general or constitutional nature and causation of the disease, while local agents were found to play only a secondary part, as exciting causes, being incapable alone of producing true eczema. Further, the influence which local causes appear to have in the production of the disease, is sometimes very difficult, if not impossible to trace.

It remains to enter more fully and definitely into the etiology of eczema, that light may be thrown upon the treatment and prevention of the disease both as to individual attacks and recurrences.

As in other diseases, we may consider the etiology of eczema under the two heads of predisposing and exciting causes; this division applies both to general or constitutional conditions, and to local agents.

The first general predisposing cause to be considered is that of constitution, or in other words, the hereditary character of the disease. In a preceding chapter, (page 17), it has been shown that in but a very small proportion of the cases, even in the higher ranks of private practice, can any strong evidence be adduced to show the heredity of eczema to any degree; the vast majority of cases do not exhibit this feature. Considering the great frequency of the disease, a very small proportion of the relatives of the eczema patients were similarly affected, indeed almost a smaller proportion than might be naturally looked for in an equal number of persons not related to those affected with eczema.

But, on the other hand, although the disease appears to come by direct inheritance in but very few cases, it is still true that in a certain number it is seen to be hereditary, and whole families are sometimes affected, not only in one generation but in several ; and naturally such cases are more difficult of treatment, although experience shows that even heredity is not a bar to cure.

In certain cases it appears highly probable that gout in the family results in eczema in the next generation, and I have seen repeated instances where gout, eczema, and asthma alternated in various generations and branches of the family in such a manner as to lead to the conclusion that they were intimately connected, and that the state or condition of system was inherited, which produced one or the other of these diseases, according to the exciting causes present.

Scrofula or struma undoubtedly appears as a predisposing cause of eczema in the way of inheritance, quite as effectively as when existing in the individual, as will be dwelt on later. Syphilis is not known to be a predisposing or exciting cause of eczema, either by heredity, or as an acquired disease, although as a depressor of vitality it may act in a secondary manner.

Considerable difference exists in different skins in regard to the susceptibility to attacks of eczema ; in some it is of itself a light, transitory affair, easily excited and easily allayed ; in others the skin becomes greatly affected and persistently so ; while in others still no amount of local irritation suffices to induce an eczematous eruption. In general, those with light hair and complexions, are more liable to be affected than those of darker hue. Some families are more prone to skin diseases in general than are others, in them the skin as an organ appears to be weak and easily affected.

Many attempts have been made by writers in the past to define the state of system which predisposes to eczema, and the terms dartrous, arthritic, rheumic, herpetic, and scrofulous diatheses are familiar to all. Some have used only the term "eczematous diathesis," and have not attempted any further explanation. But none of these diathetic theories have received the general sanction of acceptance, and yet the impression exists everywhere that there is and must be some constitutional condition which can account for the presence and continuance, often for long periods, of this rebellious disease, eczema. It must be acknowledged, however, that the true nature of the systemic changes which produce the disease has as yet eluded scientific definition; it has not been demonstrated by the microscope, test-tube, or the retort, and probably never will be.

This constitutional state is not represented by any one single, definite condition; there is no dyscrasia proper to eczema, as far as can be determined at present, although for convenience the term eczematous diathesis may perhaps best represent the totality of systemic conditions which are found in subjects of eczema; there is, however, no real foundation which is incontestable to support the existence of any such peculiar diathesis, and, if used, the expression must be taken in its broadest sense, to express a state of system whose exact components escape our observation, but whose clinical features are constantly exhibited.

Eczema is certainly not a contagious disease, it is never acquired by contact or by the introduction of any

poison from without, nor can it be produced by artificial in-
oculation. It is not conveyed in the process of vaccination
and cannot be communicated in any way, even to those
having the most intimate associations with those affected.

Notwithstanding the fact, however, that authorities
differ as to the real elements which are to be considered
causative of eczema, and notwithstanding the fact that
no single principle, such as contagion or infection, cold
or heat, or diet or occupation, can be definitely stated to
be the invariable cause of eczema, we are still in a position to define with a tolerable degree of certainty what
agencies have been shown by experience to be closely
associated with the production of attacks of eczema, and
what elements require to be removed by proper management in order to benefit or cure the disease. In other
words, we must turn from the laboratory to the sick room,
and study causes on the patient and not on paper, clinically and not theoretically.

Careful and repeated study and observation of patients with eczema will always reveal that they are not in
perfect health : sometimes the difficulty is very evident,
at other times the departure from health can only be
learned after searching investigation. But I repeat, that
eczema is not a purely local disease of the skin tissue, it
is not merely a perverted mode of action of the cells of
some particular part, but has its origin in other or constitutional relations or conditions ; although, in any one
particular case these causative conditions may have
passed away spontaneously or under treatment, while the
local *product of disease*, the thickening and infiltration of
tissue, with the consequent itching, fissures, etc., may remain, and may be amenable to purely local treatment.

This constitutional state, which may be discovered to
a greater or less degree in eczema patients, is one of debility, or lowered vitality of the whole system, or of one

or more portions ; it is one characterized by the imperfect performance of the life processes, either in the organs or systems specially charged with the supply of fresh material and the removal of effete products, or in the tissues of the body in general, including the skin.

The pulse of patients with eczema rarely represents that of health, and may be variously abnormal. It may be very sluggish in those of bilious state, and I have observed it below fifty in the minute, rising to normal frequency when this condition was removed. Far more frequently it is found to be unnaturally frequent, and may range very high from debility or neurasthenia, gradually returning to a standard of health under the treatment which cures the eczema. It is almost always weaker and more compressible than in perfect health, although occasionally in apparently robust subjects, especially in more acute cases, it may seem to be full, and may even be throbbing. In these latter cases this is found to be the result of an unnatural heart stimulation by an overloading of the circulation with effete products, resulting from imperfect assimilation and disintegration ; under a little laxative and diuretic treatment, suitable for the eczema, this full condition of the pulse ceases and the true condition of more or less weakness and compressibility is observed. Patients exhibiting this condition of the circulatory system are not infrequently the subjects of palpitation, and often of irregularities and intermissions of the pulse.

Three classes of subjects will present themselves with eczema ; or rather, most eczema patients or their families may be divided into three tolerably distinct classes. These are, first, those presenting the gouty state ; second, those exhibiting some of the elements grouped under and known as scrofula or struma, which for convenience will be spoken of as the strumous state ; and third, those manifesting symptoms more particularly referable to the nervous system, which is commonly spoken of as the neurotic state. It is by no means asserted that hard and fast lines can always be drawn, and that every one out of each hundred eczema patients can be at once placed in one group or the other; on the contrary the border lines between them are not very sharply drawn in many cases, and not at all infrequently it will be most difficult to determine clearly where some particular patient is to be located: especially do the first and third classes touch one another.

The value of recognizing these three states rests entirely on the purely practical basis of therapeutics and prophylaxis, and in this light we will study them. The relations of these three states to eczema, have been stated thus by Mr. Wilson.* "Constitutional debility may present itself in three forms; namely, as an *assimilative debility*, in which the organs of digestion and secretion are principally at fault; as a *nutritive debility*, wherein the powers of nutrition are chiefly concerned; and, as *nervous debility*, in which a morbid state of the nervous system takes the lead." The first of these classes represents that which we shall consider as the gouty state, for reasons which will appear later; this form of assimilative debility is exhibited in by far the larger share of the cases of eczema. The other forms spoken of by Mr. Wilson, namely, nutritive and nervous debility, correspond with the clinical divisions of the strumous and nervous states or types. As remarked before, these are not sharply defined conditions which can be determined with absolute accuracy in every case, but rather indicate the general directions in which investigation must turn, and toward which treatment must be directed. We will, however, treat of them separately.

To a proper understanding of what is implied by the

* Diseases of the Skin. Sixth edition; London: 1867. p. 157

influence of the "gouty state" in eczema, it will be well
first to define what is understood by this term.   When
gout is spoken of, the unprofessional mind has at once
suggested to it an exceedingly painful inflammation of
one or more of the smaller joints of the extremities, notably that of the great toe.   The physician who has given
but little thought or study to the matter, at once recalls
that gout may affect any of the organs of the body—that
there may be gout of the kidney, heart, liver, brain, etc.
He who has gone somewhat more deeply into the subject recognizes that these are all but the phenomena resulting from a blood alteration which has been demonstrated, and that the presence of uric acid in the blood
is the root of the evil, the attempted oxidation of which
in the tissues gives rise to the local inflammations.

But if the phenomena of gout are not studied or observed further even than this, we will fail to note the
connection which exists between the gouty state of which
we speak, and functional and other diseases of the system,
as eczema.   The true student of the gouty state must
enter deeper into its pathology than the simple existence
of the inflammation of the joints, or of the internal organs
of the body, and even deeper than the acid-blood state
which is recognized as the foundation of these ; he must
seek for the causes of this state of the blood ; he must
search for the earlier manifestations of the blood alteration, which may be discovered a great while before the
joints or viscera are inflamed or altered ; he must recognize the elements which form the beginning of the long
train of cause and effect which eventuates, if its course
is unchecked or unchanged, in what is commonly known
as gouty inflammation.   The earlier links in the chain
are quite as important as the later, or rather are much
more important therapeutically, inasmuch as it is during
this period that, by proper regulation of the patient's

life, with slight medication, or by the "management of the gouty state," we may do much to avert an evil which will surely come if the earlier warnings of greater or less severity are not heeded and acted upon in time. It is in this light that I look upon many of the cutaneous and mucous inflammations which often long precede the commonly recognized symptoms of gout, and very prominent among these stands eczema, in very many instances.

I confess that I cannot understand how this influence could have been so overlooked as it has been by local pathologists, for surely a careful study of recorded private cases in sufficient numbers cannot fail to convince the most skeptical of a very frequent co-existence of eczema and the phenomena now recognized by the best authorities as gouty, and a careful following out of the cases on paper, day by day, certainly shows that as • one set of symptoms improves the others commonly do the same, and *vice versa;* and that remedies affecting the one are of influence over the other.

Turning now to the more immediate consideration of the subject, what are the elements comprising the gouty state which we are to seek for and recognize as of importance in connection with eczema? They may be classed under two heads; imperfect assimilation, and imperfect disassimilation or disintegration. By these two processes growth and repair are carried on and effete products removed; failure in one or both of these involves failure in the processes of life and health. The clinical signs by which these are manifested are, imperfect digestion, constipation and diarrhœa, imperfect urinary secretion, and faulty cutaneous action.

Imperfect digestion, indigestion, or dyspepsia, represents a failure in the process of preparation and assimilation of the food by the various organs, alone or com-

bined, which are charged with the function of ministering to the nutrition of the body. In the cases here
analyzed the various phases of indigestion were met with
to a degree of frequency which would surprise one unfamiliar with the subject.

If patients with eczema are asked whether they have
any indigestion, a considerable number will state that
they have not, although some proportion will say that
they have, meaning thereby that they suffer from some
of the forms of primary indigestion which obtrude themselves in ways which are decidedly uncomfortable. Thus,
the most commonly recognized symptoms of dyspepsia,
such as, pain after eating or the feeling of a heavy load
in the stomach, heart-burn, nausea, acrid or fetid eructations of fluid or wind, are familiar to many, and may or
may not be mentioned by the patient if they exist.

But it is a mistake to suppose if these are absent that
the patient may not have imperfect digestion, and it has
been the failure to recognize this fact and to search for
deeper proof which has led to many mistakes and failures
in the management of eczema. Imperfect digestion is
shown quite as plainly by other signs than those recognized by the laity, and if these are sought for they
will often be found in eczema patients.

These signs of imperfect digestion have been very
carefully studied by the late Dr. Murchison, and many
of them referred by him, very reasonably, to functional
derangement of the liver. His observations have been
so continually verified in my practice that I shall avail
myself of his clear and definite statements in regard to
many points. The following list of symptoms representing this state is adapted from his excellent Croonian
Lectures on Functional Derangements of the Liver.

1. A feeling of weight and fullness at the epigastrium,
and in the region of the liver.

2. Flatulent distension of the stomach and bowels.

3. Heart-burn and acid eructations.

4. A feeling of oppression and often of weariness, and aching pains in the limbs, or of insurmountable sleepiness after meals.

5. A furred tongue, which is often large and indented at the edges, and a clammy, bitter, or metallic taste in the mouth, especially in the morning.

6. Appetite often good: at other times anorexia and nausea.

7. An excessive secretion of viscid mucus in the fauces and at the back of the nose.

8. Constipation, the motions being scybalous, sometimes too dark, at others too light, or even clay-colored; occasionally attacks of diarrhœa alternating with constipation, especially if the patient is intemperate in the use of alcohol.

9. In some patients attacks of palpitation of the heart, or irregularity or intermission of the pulse.

10. In many patients occasional attacks of frontal headache.

11. In many patients restlessness at night and bad dreams.

12. In some patients attacks of vertigo or dimness of sight, often induced by particular articles of diet.

To these may be added other signs more or less marked, such as: a slow and sluggish pulse; chronic bronchitis and spasmodic asthma; aphthous sores of the mouth and tongue; hemorrhoidal congestion, with external or internal piles, and pruritus of the anus; a dry or parched state of the tongue and mouth in the night or on awaking; and a want of refreshment in sleep, the patient often feeling more tired on rising than on going to bed.

Not infrequently almost the sole sign of mal-assimilation which attracts attention is a great lassitude, and indisposition to any work, either mental or physical, and continually during the treatment of eczema by proper medication, diet, etc., will one hear the statement that the patient who before felt indisposed to any exertion now feels a freshness and vigor of life which had not been experienced perhaps for months or even years.

Such are many of the states which may constantly be observed in patients with eczema, although often many of them seem to be absent, and often they are discovered only after careful search. Some of these may be considered a little more in detail.

The causes of this imperfect digestion are manifold, and need not be entered upon here; they are such as pertain to the various derangements incident to life. Prominent among these is wrong eating and insufficient oxidation by means of fresh air and exercise. There can be little doubt in the mind of the intelligent observer, that among those who are able to obtain the necessities and luxuries of life a larger number of persons over-eat than take less than the necessities of life and activity demand; while the amount of physical exercise in the fresh air sufficient to give life and vigor to the frame, is seldom taken. This increase of material over the amount required, combined with a diminished activity to consume that taken, results in a loading of the system with the products of imperfect assimilation and disintegration, and produces the accompanying train of ill feelings manifested in the most varied manner in the different organs of the body. If the stomach is taxed just a little beyond its capability it must either reject the surplus or pass the whole mass on to other organs in an imperfectly elaborated manner. The liver is then not only presented with rather more material than it is really capable of caring for, but it has to do its work upon a substance which the stomach has not quite prepared for its action. The same is true of the pancreas and the intestines, and when in the course of the circulation the imperfectly digested material and poorly elaborated blood comes to the lungs, they have not only the same extra amount of food to care for, just a little above their normal quota, but they have a blood to aërate which has received partially digested elements ; and, when the kidneys attempt to filter off the excrementitious portions which they naturally select, they do not find the urea ready for them, but the other elements in the form of uric acid in combination, and oxalate of lime, or perhaps sugar, or even albumen.

The skin must share in this train of evil results, and its glands cannot elaborate their proper substances from a blood supply which has been imperfectly prepared; and it is as yet impossible to tell how large a share this failure in the perfect action of the cutaneous glands may have to do with many of the lesions of this great organ, whose daily excretion is almost equal to that of the lungs or kidneys.

This is no idle picture, but is one from nature, one of daily occurrence, and one which cannot be disproved, or disregarded.

But not only do the various organs ministering to nutrition suffer, from being unable to perform their functions properly, so that in almost all of those mentioned we may and do often have pain or various ill feelings as indications of their imperfect action, but we have also symptoms coming from still other organs, and even from any or every portion of the body. With a blood current already filled with the elements of imperfect assimilation we cannot have a perfect and thorough absorption or taking up of effete materials from the tissues, or perfect disassimilation. The brain and nerves then indicate their inadequate supply of proper material

and their overloading with effete matter by pain, and
we have the various phenomena of sick headache and
neuralgias of different regions. Or, the brain manifests
its uneasiness by restlessness in sleep or by troublesome
or terrifying dreams ; by sleepiness after eating, and
wakefulness at the proper time of sleep ; or by inability
to perform mental work, peevishness or depression of
spirits, etc.

The muscles show their mal-nutrition by a sense of
fatigue and indisposition to the very exertion which is
needed to quicken the circulation and hasten the processes of life, or by aching or twitchings. The heart
muscle does its work spasmodically, and we have palpi-
tations, or very frequent pulsations ; or, sometimes a
very slow beat with, occasionally, omissions. The lungs
also show signs of their suffering, in sighing respiration,
and occasional attacks of spasmodic or asthmatic breathing ; while all the upper mucous passages give rise to
augmented secretion with each occurrence of imperfect
digestion, a state familiar to all as catarrh of various
regions. This latter may become continuous when the
system is continually subjected to these results of partially elaborated food supply and partially removed effete
material. Other mucous surfaces may also suffer, and
we have leucorrhœa, etc., as a common accompaniment
of eczema.

No one who has been a careful observer of cases of
chronic disease can fail to recognize in this picture the
state which is so often found in those with gouty antecedents or gouty tendencies of their own. Sooner or
later this train of phenomena leads to deterioration and
disorganization of some organ or organs. With these
products of imperfect nutrition circulating in the blood
giving rise to irritation of tissue, we very readily have
local inflammations. The joint of the large toe, one of

the most frequently used joints in the body, and one constantly subjected to pressure and to occasional injury, besides being the joint furthest from the centre of circulation, becomes inflamed and we have what is then recognized by all as gout. But the patient had gout long before the inflammation came on ; and he has the gouty state if chance should cause some other accident, and if some other portion of the body, such as kidneys, lungs, etc., should become inflamed, from a capillary stasis of this blood, overladen with effete products and with particles not in a condition from which healthy tissue can be formed.

Some local agent causes the skin of a certain portion to become irritated and inflamed, and here may be gout of the skin just as surely as we have had gout of the fibrous and synovial portions of the joints. This is then the constitutional element which requires to be met in many cases of eczema.

Constipation is found to be a most frequent accompaniment of eczema, as shown in the cases here analyzed ; and so constantly is the eruption benefited to a greater or less degree by its removal, that we must look upon an imperfect bowel secretion and excretion as an important factor in the genesis of eczema.

There are undoubtedly many forms of torpidity of the intestinal functions, and they are due to many different causes ; but the fact remains, that imperfect removal from the system of those elements which should be excreted through the intestine is a source of the aggravation of eczema, if it be not an efficient cause of the disease. The subject of constipation from nervous or general debility, or from the repeated neglect of the calls of nature, or from the constant and frequent abuse of purgatives or enemata, cannot be fully discussed here ; the variety of trouble must be studied out and remedied, and that not by spasmodic stimulation with drastic or saline cathartics, but by a careful remedying of the cause and the installation of a regular, satisfactory, and sufficient, discharge of normal fæcal matter from the bowels. This will often prove a very difficult task, but it is worth the effort both of the patient and physician. For a full discussion of constipation, the reader is referred to the excellent little book of Dr. Birch, on Constipated Bowels, which contains very much common sense which should be put in daily practice.

Another mode in which the imperfect carrying out of the processes of life is manifested, is in the altered condition of the urinary secretion. This does not refer to organic kidney disease, for most commonly the disorder is but functional, and the urinary error is not so much the fault of the kidney, as it is of the state of the blood current and the organs on which this depends.

These changes of course are not always manifest on casual observation, or learned from brief inquiry of the patient, but like the other elements of this state of imperfect vitalization must be sought for. Objectively we will often learn that the urine is high colored or muddy, and that on standing it deposits a pinkish or yellow sediment of urates, which stain the vessel; or, it may have the red-pepper-like crystals of uric acid; or, it may exhibit a phosphatic pellicle on the surface. Subjectively the patient may complain of burning or scalding, on micturition; or, there may be inability to hold the water, so that the frequent calls must be immediately answered, or the garments will be wet. It is not at all uncommon for children with eczema to have the habit of wetting the bed at night, or even the clothes during the day, and the same alkaline treatment which removes this yields excellent results in the eczema. Very many adults with eczema will also be found to have the habit of rising once or several times during the night, for the purpose of emptying the bladder ; this also improves, or is often entirely removed as the eczema state subsides under proper treatment. Again, many patients will pass very large quantities of limpid urine, or will themselves notice that that voided at one time of day is quite different from that at another hour.

But often the patient will report nothing wrong with the urine, and yet examination will show it to be far from normal. Albumen and sugar are not common, though they are sometimes found transiently, even in those without chronic albuminuria or glycosuria. The presence of these substances will generally be found to be associated with some error of diet, or from over-indulgence in sugar or albumen. The specific gravity will be found to vary most markedly in eczema, ranging, from 1,030 down to as low as 1,004, and not infrequently that passed on retiring will give a high specific gravity, while the urine of rising will have a very low gravity. Oxalate of lime is a pretty constant deposit in the urine of patients with eczema of any extent or severity, and urates and uric acid may often be seen microscopically when hardly suspected from ordinary inspection.

The second causative influence which is found in a certain proportion of cases of eczema must be recognized in that illy defined but still practically acknowledged condition or state called scrofula or struma. No one can see much of public practice without discovering a certain class of patients to whom the term strumous or scrofulous is given almost instinctively, without particular thought as to the elements composing the state in question. These subjects present the pale, delicate skin, sometimes almost translucent, with brilliancy of color on excitement, and soft, fine, and generally light colored hair.

Or, the complexion may be pasty, thick, and coarse, with a thick and prominent upper lip. Such subjects are very liable to affections of the mucous membranes, as chronic nasal catarrh, otorrhœa, and chronic inflammation of the eyes, frequently leaving corneal opacities; the abdomen is swollen, the head large, and the muscles are small and flabby. Disease of the bones readily occurs, and the lymphatics become enlarged, and some glands can usually be felt, if indeed they do not suppurate, leaving ugly cicatrices.

As with the gouty state, previously described, an accurate description of the strumous constitution or habit is extremely difficult, and the condition has not been and probably never will be demonstrated absolutely by any of the exact methods of science. But clinically such a state exists and exerts a great influence upon eczema; indeed, it has long been acknowledged by many authorities as one of the causative elements of the disease.

The eruption of eczema in a marked case of the gouty state and the same eruption in a strumous case present all the differences imaginable; in the latter the tendency to the production of pus is striking, and if the lesions do not assume the form of a distinct impetiginous eczema, the crusts which form are yellow and thick, and the quantity of pus is entirely disproportionate to the intensity of the inflammation; indeed, the entire picture contrasts strongly with the red, highly inflamed surface of the gouty form, with its thin, glairy secretion drying into lighter, whiter scales.

The exact bearing which this strumous state has upon the production of eczema cannot be stated, but as a sign of debility and as an indication for a particular line of treatment, it should never fail to be recognized when present. Neumann states that about one third of the eczematous children which he examined in reference to this point were found to be rachitic or scrofulous, and Wilson gives a somewhat larger proportion as exhibiting nutritive debility. I regret that I have not kept statistics in full in reference to this point, but am fully impressed with the clinical existence of the strumous state in eczema patients and of its important bearing in producing the disease. It is true that we do not very often see the late manifestations of the diathesis, as caries of the bones, or even suppurating glands or phthisis, in immediate connection with eczema; but the same holds true with the strumous which has been stated of the gouty state, namely, that we are to recognize the earlier manifestations rather than to wait till the later are apparent; the inflammatory skin lesions belong to a period before the inflammation of the joints occurs in the one, or disease of the bones and caseous deposits in the other.

It is not at all uncommon to find eczema associated with ulceration of the cornea, and the tendency to boils and carbuncles so frequently exhibited by eczema patients points in the direction of a strumous habit. It must not be forgotten that this strumous or scrofulous condition can exist in adults and even in the aged, although it is far more commonly spoken of as belonging to childhood; the lowered vitality which marks this state in the young and gives rise to the pale and pasty skin, flabby muscles, and the ready formation of pus, may continue even to advanced age, and undoubtedly influences to a greater or less degree all the processes of health and disease.

The third condition or habit which is of clinical importance etiologically in many cases of eczema is the neurotic state. This appears to be of comparatively little influence in children, but in adults it is frequently of the very greatest significance; nervous debility is an element which is daily being recognized more and more, and neurasthenia has a train of symptoms which pertain to most of the organs of the body, and often strikingly to the skin.

In the chapter upon the symptoms of eczema, and its anatomy, the subject of the nerve relations of the disease was fully treated of as far as physiological and pathological researches were concerned, and it was found that they were of no mean importance in the production of the eruption. The first and most prominent symptom in eczema was stated to be the itching, or, a burning pain in the more acute forms, which often occurs before an eruption is seen, and also after external signs have quite disappeared. It remains now to study the subject more closely from a clinical standpoint.

If we were to regard as neurotic only those patients who in themselves or their immediate family exhibited the grosser and more severe forms of disease commonly spoken of as nervous, such as brain and spinal disease, or even chorea, epilepsy, or hysteria, we would, as in the case of the gouty and strumous state, fall far short of a proper comprehension of the relations which neurasthenia bears to eczema. It is not the graver manifestations which mark the diathesis or state, but rather the grouping of corroborative symptoms which shows the tendency or direction in which the current of life tends.

Nervous debility, neurasthenia, or lowered vitality of nerve action, is frequently observed in eczema patients of young and middle life in private practice, and requires to be recognized and met in order to a successful management of the case. Not at all infrequently this neurotic state will have been induced by prolonged assimilative disorder, or the gouty state, but it will also often be the direct result of nervous overstrain, and sometimes of shock.

This portion of the subject, which is a very difficult one, cannot be better developed and demonstrated than by the brief mention of a few instances, out of many, which have appeared to be most striking. Miss D., aged 53, was the executive officer of a charitable institution. Her Tuesday's work of each week was very severe and trying, on account of the weekly meeting of and inspection by the board of lady visitors; and that night was often sleepless. Her eczema of the face and hands was always greatly aggravated on the succeeding morning; often, indeed, the eczema, which would almost yield to treatment during the interval, would burst out afresh on the Wednesday morning succeeding the visit. This had been the case for some months before I saw her, and was verified by myself time and again. Rev. Dr. B., a prominent clergyman aged 52, had for many years an eczema of the head and face which was always immensely aggravated on Monday, after the Sabbath's mental work and strain. The same occurred whenever extra work, as public addresses, etc., was called for. Mrs. M., aged 32, a widow, who used the hand very greatly in writing for the press, and was also subject to very great nervous overstrain as editor of a department in a weekly journal, had an eruption of papular eczema over the right shoulder and following the nerve tracts down the arm. Whenever rest was given to the arm, that is abstinence from writing, the disease yielded readily, but the eruption would return in the same location whenever exhaustion was reached. She was a perfect type of a neurotic female, having had paralysis herself and having insanity in the family. Electricity in the form of central galvanization gave her great relief. In another case, that of a lady aged 22, each nervous excitement, as hysterical crying or household disturbance, would be followed by a fresh outburst of eczema on the hands.

These illustrations could be multiplied very greatly; in scores of cases I have found the nervous element to be of the greatest importance, and if we cannot speak of the neurotic state as an efficient cause for eczema in certain cases, there is nothing true in clinical medicine.

In the table giving the ages of all cases of eczema, (page 12), we find the number of cases in males between the ages of 10 and 20 years, to be 105 ; between 20 and 30 years the number is exactly doubled, namely 210, while between 30 and 40 years of age, it runs up to 250 cases. That is, during the period between 20 and 40 years of life, when the nervous strain comes on men, the total number of cases was 460, or nearly one-third of all the cases in males. This is shown still more strikingly in Table II., from private practice, where, with 34 cases observed between 10 and 20 years of age, we have 90, or almost three times as many between 20 and 30, and 153 cases between the ages of 30 and 40 years.

In regard to the manner in which this nervous influence operates, we can only conjecture. But it seems probable that there are several modes in which the nervous debility or depression can produce its results, as was mentioned in a previous chapter, (page 32.) First, by a direct effect upon the cells, whereby the life process is altered, and a disease process or inflammation takes its place. Second, through the agency of the vasomotor nerves, altering the nutrition of the part by means of the blood supply. Third, in an indirect manner through the scratching, etc., induced by the itching ; and, Fourth, in another secondary manner through the agency of the digestion. All are familiar with the power of fright and grief in arresting the processes of digestion, and it is more than probable that much of the effect produced ordinarily by lowered nervous vitality relates to

digestive and assimilative disorders, which in their turn
provoke the eczema.

The symmetry which is so frequently exhibited to a
striking degree in eczema, might be regarded, and rightly,
as an evidence of nervous relations of the disease. As
before shown, in by far the larger share of instances, the
eruption appears without any discernible local cause ;
upon protected parts especially a symmetrical disposition may be very commonly traced to such a degree as
to be most striking, and often the distribution is found
to correspond very closely to definite nerve tracts. No
entirely satisfactory demonstration or explanation of the
neurotic relations of eczema can be yet made out, but in
the light of present knowledge sufficient is determined
to show the importance of considering this element in
the management of the disease.

We have thus far considered only the predisposing
causes of eczema of internal or constitutional origin.
We have found that there was certainly no single definite cause, no *materies morbi* seeking exit through the
skin, whose presence caused the eruption, but that debility in some of its forms was at the bottom of the
disease.

Besides the predisposing causes of internal or constitutional origin, we have also certain others which may
be regarded as exciting internal causes.

When treating of the gouty state, dyspepsia and imperfect intestinal excretion were spoken of as factors of
great importance. These same elements must now be
mentioned as sources of fresh attacks or exacerbations
of the disease ; that is, fresh or increased digestive disorder can, and very frequently does, excite fresh outbreaks of the cutaneous lesion ; this will be especially
alluded to in connection with eczema of the face, hands,

and arms. Renewed constipation also serves to excite afresh an eruption which may have slumbered long, or may retard an improvement which had previously progressed satisfactorily.

Menstrual difficulties must be recognized as a cause of eczema, and in many cases the eruption is decidedly worse with the occurrence of each monthly flow; where there is rebellious menorrhagia or dysmenorrhœa, the eczema often proves most intractable. In what manner disturbances of the sexual organs act to predispose to, or to excite an eczema cannot be stated, but the observation may be made clinically, that an intimate relation often exists between uterine or ovarian derangement and the eruption of eczema.

Statistics also show that the menses have some influence in eczema. Thus in Table I., it will be seen that the number of males and females were almost equal during the first ten years of life, whereas in the period of the establishment of the menses, between ten and twenty years, the females were in the great majority, forming 64.16 per cent of all the cases.

The meno-pause is supposed to have an effect in causing the appearance of eczema, and statistics show this also to a certain degree. Thus in the table alluded to, we find that between the ages of 30 and 40, there were 166 females affected with eczema, whereas, between 40 and 50 years of age, the period during which the cessation of the menses is looked for, there were 188 cases, while in the next decade there occurred but 137 cases. Among the males for the same period, there were 250 cases between 30 and 40 years of age, 214 between 40 and 50, and 196 between 50 and 60 years.

Pregnancy is recognized as a cause of the appearance of eczema by several writers, and Hebra even states that some women are more sure of impregnation from the occurrence of eczema of the hands than from any other symptom. I have seen many cases of eczema in pregnant women, but could never satisfy myself of any causative influence, and have seen many cases of eczema cured during the continuance of the pregnancy.

Lactation is undoubtedly an exciting cause in some instances, but it is questionable if it ever operates in any other manner than by causing the debility which results in the disease.

Dentition is beyond question a fruitful cause of the eruption of eczema, as any one who has seen many cases of this disease in infants must acknowledge ; for continually we observe a fresh accession of the eruption with the irruption of each tooth. In Table I, it will be seen that considerably more than three-quarters of all the cases in the first decade of life, occurred during the first three years. But it will also be shown later that this is not a necessary cause, since in multitudes of infants the eruption is cured during dentition. It is doubtful whether this acts more than as a disturber of digestion, although it is more than probable that there is also some effect produced through the agency of the nervous system ; as we know that the nerve disturbance consequent on dentition is often very considerable.

The irritation produced by the presence of intestinal worms may occasionally be an exciting cause of eczema. Stricture of the urethra is asserted by Anderson to excite the eruption in certain cases, and I have met with one instance which seemed to demonstrate this, and believe it quite possible.

Varicose veins are a prolific source of eczema of the lower extremities, and often render the disease in this situation most difficult of cure. The slowness of the circulation in the parts, consequent upon the enlargement of the area of the veins, gives ready cause for the exudation of fluid, while it hinders the absorption of effete matter by the capillaries and lymphatics.

Certain chronic disease states are sometimes thought to have a bearing upon the etiology of eczema, such as chronic disease of the kidneys and heart, diabetes, etc. I have never been able to satisfy myself as to any connection of this kind ; among many hundred examinations of the urine of eczema patients it has been the rarest event to find organic disease of the kidneys, and among many patients with Bright's disease seen in hospital practice, eczema was very rarely observed. Nor has organic heart disease been observed to be thus connected. I have not infrequently seen diabetes mellitus associated with eczema ; but in these cases the eruption begins about the genitals, following the scratching to relieve itching there. Other points bearing on this subject have been generally considered in the second chapter, toward its close.

We come now to speak of the local causes of eczema, which by some are exalted into a much greater prominence than is here assigned to them. Careful observation and study of the cases upon which this work is based (and some of the cases have extended over years with many relapses at longer or shorter intervals), have convinced me that altogether too much stress has been laid upon external agencies, as causes of the disease, or even as excitants of the eruption at any particular time and place. I have searched in vain for the operation of the various irritants named in the books, more especially among intelligent patients in private practice, and have to say that in the vast proportion of instances I have not been able to discover any local cause which would account for the existence or continuance of the eruption. And on the contrary we see any number of individuals exposed to a greater or less amount of local irritation who escape all skin lesions, or if inflammation is produced it appears only as a transient dermatitis.

which should be carefully differentiated from true eczema. And, as alluded to in a previous chapter (page 81), we often see the same person exposed to a cutaneous irritant for a long time, without developing an eczema, until finally under a depression of health or some general cause the skin becomes affected; and then the eruption will often occur in some remote part as well as in that exposed to the injurious irritant.

The external agent to which I would give first place as a cause of eczema is the atmospheric condition, notwithstanding the fact that Hebra ridicules the idea that "catching cold" can be regarded as an etiological factor in eczema. What the exact relations of the disease to climatic changes are I cannot at present say, but that in one way or another atmospheric influences produce, excite, and prolong eczema I am confident.

Eczema patients are as a class unusually susceptible to the cold, and many are even better barometers than are confirmed rheumatics : each change in the weather can either be foretold or tells its own story in the condition of the skin. This, of course cannot be demonstrated in every case, and in infants it might readily be overlooked, but if these cases are carefully watched fresh outbreaks will often be seen to follow outdoor exposure.

It is not the cold alone which is injurious to eczema, nor great heat, although we must acknowledge with writers that these are efficient exciting causes of the eruption in many cases. But it appears to be the humidity of the atmosphere and possibly its ozonic condition, which has the prejudicial effect on the disease ; accurate observations are much needed in this direction. Eczema appears to be most frequent along the sea coast and in moist climates, and most cases of eczema are made worse at the sea shore.

In regard to the effect of the season of the year upon the production of eczema it is difficult to form any accurate conclusions, statements of patients often appear to be very contradictory. It may be stated that in public practice a larger number of infants are affected in summer, than during other seasons, from the results of the heat, while in private practice adults exhibit eczema much more in winter than in summer. It is exceedingly common to hear that the eruption reappears or is aggravated with the beginning of the cold weather, while in many instances it disappears spontaneously in a warm and equable climate.

That undefined and undefinable process of "catching cold," most certainly has much to do with the genesis and continuance of eczema, and a check of perspiration or chilling of the surface will constantly be followed by aggravation of the disease.

The next agency external to the person which operates to cause eczema is occupation, and this is a subject fraught with very considerable interest in regard to the etiology of the disease. Occupation may act prejudicially in two ways, first by deteriorating the health, as by confinement in bad air, and by sedentary habits; and second by furnishing the direct local causes for exciting the outbreak of the eruption. Sedentary pursuits are far more conducive to the disease than even those involving considerable exposure. A sudden change from an active life to one requiring confinement to the house may readily result in the development of the eczema state. Business demanding much nervous strain conduces to the disease, also one which subjects the individual to irregularity in living. Vocations which require much standing still are very apt to cause eczema of the lower limbs from the impeded circulation. Thus we see eczema of the legs in type setters, cooks, wood turners, car drivers and others, generally accompanied by varicose veins.

The local agents which may operate to cause eczema during occupation, are as numerous as are the irritants which can inflame or destroy living tissues ; there is nothing peculiar to be stated in reference to them. A few of the more important may be here mentioned; these and others will be more particularly alluded to in connection with eczema of various localities.

Cooks and laundresses may have eczema of the face and hands from the fire, or of the hands and arms from the constant action of the water, and the soap and alkalies used, combined with the effects of heat. Masons, plasterers and bricklayers have eczema from the lime, and bakers from the flour, likewise grocers from the substances handled. Workers in various chemical substances, dyers, hat-finishers, and others may have an eczema started from an irritant used in manufacture.

The local irritant may come in many and often unexpected ways. Burns are sometimes followed by eczema, also the application of irritants which are harmless to many skins. Poison ivy (Rhus toxicodendron) and also poison sumach may give rise to a persistent eczema, although the dermatitis occasioned thereby usually passes off quickly and leaves no trace. Various dyes, especially those produced by aniline colors, will occasion very severe eczema in those predisposed to the disease, and stockings, gloves, undershirts, and even hat-bands will give rise to it, as I have repeatedly seen.

Substances used in medicine may also have this effect, and the external use of arnica has frequently been followed by intense inflammation of the skin, resulting in eczema. The same is true to a less degree of cantharides, capsicum, thapsia, mezereon, tartar emetic, croton-oil, chrysophanic acid, and even mustard. Sulphur ointment, used for the treatment of scabies will sometimes excite an undue amount of inflammation which may result in eczema ; and not infrequently the papular eruption caused by the application will be mistaken for an increase of the original trouble, and the remedy will be pushed, only to the aggravation of the condition. Mercurial inunctions will also sometimes inflame the skin very considerably.

What has been spoken of as mercurial eczema by older writers, is probably only the local inflammation which is occasionally quite severe, from the application of mercurial ointment in the course of inunctions for syphilis; an eruption caused by the internal administration of mercury is exceedingly rare, if it ever occurs, and never takes a form resembling eczema.

The irritating effects of harsh soaps, also that of shaving, must not be forgotten; likewise, the local irritation of combing the scalp to remove dandruff or pediculi. Irritating underclothing, even though it contain no dye, sometimes gives rise to an eczematous eruption, as is occasionally seen at the beginning of winter; also chafing of the parts about the folds, at the genital region and under the breasts, together with the irritating secretions and moisture retained there, sometimes give rise to very intractable eczema both in children and adults.

Scratching the skin to relieve the itching of any eruption, urticaria, pruritus and prurigo, etc, may also excite eczema, in proper subjects; most of the lesions seen in scabies and pediculosis are due to the scratching employed, and in eczematous subjects may go on to the development of eczema. Likewise the itching of a very mild eczema, long before or after there are any lesions on the skin, may give rise to a severe eruption, if the desire to scratch is greatly yielded to. Surgical dressings may excite an eruption of eczema in one predisposed thereto.

But, as stated before, in a very large share of the cases of eczema, it is absolutely impossible to discover the local cause, indeed the eruption seems to burst out in such an unaccountable way as to well support the ancient notion which gave us the terms "eruption" and "eczema," signifying to burst out and to boil over. It is, therefore, to the internal causes or states that we are especially to look, while we are most careful to remove external causes as far as possible.

But, still further, it is quite often the ordinary occupation which has apparently caused the eruption, and it is necessary that the patient should continue this if possible. And we constantly do see those who have eczema, as cooks, house servants, and others who are able to return to irritating occupations and yet keep free from the eruption. The highest art of medicine seeks to accomplish this, and this end will be best attained by paying most attention to general causes and conditions.

There are a few other factors which have been considered by writers to be of etiological importance in eczema, which may be briefly mentioned in this connection.

The exanthematous eruptions have been supposed to predispose to eczema by their effect in weakening the skin tissue. I have never been able to verify this in the slightest degree, indeed I have seen so very many infants with eczema who have not yet experienced any of these affections, and again, of the multitudes attacked by these contagious diseases so few are affected with eczema, certainly within any reasonable period of time thereafter, that I cannot assign to them any causative effect worthy of practical consideration.

Vaccination has been stated by some to be a cause of eczema, and undoubtedly cases are observed from time to time where this eruption has followed the operation of vaccination, perhaps immediately. But that it cannot be looked upon as more than an ordinary skin irritant, giving the starting point for the inflammation of the skin, in a predisposed subject, must be granted in consideration of facts similar to those alluded to in reference to the exanthemata; namely, that many infants have eczema before

vaccination is practiced, and that on the other hand, with
the almost universal practice of vaccination the operation
is followed very rarely by an immediate attack of eczema,
if, indeed, the eruption appears at all. Again it is my constant practice to allow unprotected eczema patients to be
vaccinated, even during the existence of the disease, provided it be not too acute, without any deleterious effect. I
once applied the vaccine matter directly to a raw eczematous surface, with no other denudation, on the left arm of
an infant who had not yet been vaccinated ; the virus
took, a vesicle was formed and ran a rather protracted
course, causing considerable inflammation to the adjoining
eczematous surface; but in the end all went well, the eczema was cured by appropriate remedies, though with
some difficulty, and a vaccination scar was left. As a re-
markable commentary on the subject may be mentioned
the fact that lately vaccination has been advocated as a
cure for eczema, and cases have been reported in the journals in support of the view.

The subject of the effect of tobacco in producing or prolonging eczema is a very interesting and important one, but
one about which writers have been silent. From a number
of cases in which the connection has been very manifest,
and from very considerable attention to the subject, I am
certain that tobacco, if used at all in excess, has a most
harmful effect in eczema ; the amount which can be used,
and the degree of harmfulness rests largely on individual
peculiarities. The ill effects are produced in three ways:
first, from disturbances of the digestive system, which are
common in those using tobacco largely ; second, through
the agency of the nervous system, from the depressing
effects of the tobacco ; and, third, as far as relates to smoking, from the irritating properties of the fumes, especially upon eczema about the face and hands ; this last pertains also to snuff taking, which is happily less common.

CHAPTER VIII.

UNDERSTANDING the constitutional relations and nature of eczema, and the part which local causes play in the production of the eruption, it will be readily appreciated that the management of the disease must include both general measures and those addressed to the local state present, which we have seen to be one of inflammation, either acute or chronic. The constitutional treatment embraces diet, hygiene, and internal medication, while local treatment includes the most varied applications, protective, soothing, astringent, and stimulating, according to the nature of the case.

Diet and hygiene will be reserved for a final chapter ; internal and local treatment, as commonly understood, will be here discussed with reference to their general relations, leaving special remedies and measures, and their application, to be detailed more particularly in connection with the various forms of the disease in which they are of service.

The first fact to be remembered in the treatment of the disease is that there is not and never can be any specific for eczema, and, moreover, that there is no single remedy nor even any course or plan of treatment which will be effective in every case, nor yet in the same case under every circumstance. The disease is not always due to the same, well defined cause, and cannot always be cured or even benefited by the same remedy or measures, general or local. Arsenic is not a specific for eczema, as the practice of some would seem to indicate, indeed in many cases it is useless and unnecessary, and in many others it does actual harm.

The next point to be recognized, as shown in previous chapters, is that eczema is a disease of lowered vitality, general and local, and that the aim of treatment is to restore vital tone to the system and to the integument affected. The means employed, therefore, should not be depressing, but the tendency of the entire management should be to raise the grade of life action, from that of disease to health. This applies equally to the constitutional and local measures employed.

But the caution is here necessary against the improper use of tonic and stimulant remedies and means, both internal and external; all are not equally serviceable, nor is any particular one of value at all times. A fire may be choked when low by too large a supply of fresh coal, or by improper material; and the removal of the ashes and a proper draught are quite as important to a bright fire as is good fuel. Arsenic, iron, cod-liver-oil, quinine, alcohol, milk, beef-tea, most nourishing food, and out-door exercise are all of service in treating eczema, but may do harm if improperly used, and if the organs of digestion and the processes of assimilation and disassimilation are deranged. The same is true of stimulating local treatment which while applicable to later stages is injurious during the more acute periods.

It will be here remembered that eczema is spoken of in the sense in which it has been understood in the preceding chapters, that is, not as a local disease, a dermatitis, caused by external irritants alone, but as a definite disease state, having important, though varying connections with derangements of other organs besides the skin. It is to be also recognized, however, that eczema like urticaria, may, in certain cases, be, the result of a temporary disturbance of the system, and that the eruption may then disappear under proper local measures alone, the transitory internal cause having already passed away. But this is a matter to be appreciated and determined in each case; in the management of eczema the entire condition of the patient is to be taken into consideration and all departures from health should be looked into and rectified, as far as possible, inasmuch as any one of them may be an efficient element in prolonging the disease.

It is difficult if not impossible to separate entirely the subject of the constitutional treatment of acute eczema from that belonging to chronic states, for, according to the principles here accepted, eczema in itself tends to become a chronic disease, although the skin manifestations may be acute; the constitutional features described as belonging to eczema in general relate to cases exhibiting an acute as well as a chronic eruption, and it is largely in the local measures that the differences of management are found, as will be detailed later.

Acute eczema as a rule requires light diet, mild cathartics, and alkalies, and moderate purgation for a day or so will generally be followed by relief to the full tense feeling and diminution in the cutaneous congestion; a pill containing a little blue mass and ipecac (Formula 13), or, the compound cathartic pills of the pharmacopœia answer well, while for children calomel serves best. We may also use with advantage a mixture of sulphate of magnesium and iron (Formula 1), giving it after each meal; for a slight laxative an additional dose on rising, in one half a tumbler-full of water or more, hot or warm if it can be so taken.

For an alkali I prefer the acetate of potassium (Formula 2), and if there is inaction of the general surface of the skin and of the kidneys, I combine it with sweet spirits of nitre and spiritus Mindereri (Formula 3), and a little aconite if there is febrile action. In cases where

there is some dyspepsia, with flatulence, I prefer the rhubarb and soda mixture (Formula 7), alone, or containing
in addition sulphate of magnesium or acetate of potassium.
Arsenic is not of service in an acute eczematous eruption,
but generally does harm. When acute attacks or exacerbations occur during the course of chronic eczema, it is
well to suspend the use of the arsenic, also of the more
powerful tonics, iron, etc., and to give a laxative and cooling course. The acute manifestations of eczema are
usually managed easily on the above plan, but in the sub-
acute and chronic states every resource of therapeutics
will sometimes be required for a complete and permanent
removal of the disease.

While in a previous chapter it was stated that malaria
could not be looked upon as the cause of eczema, as had
been claimed by some, it is yet very important to bear this
element in mind in the treatment of the disease ; for when
it does exist in the individual it acts as a bar to the cure
of eczema, and the preparations of cinchona often play an
important part in the treatment of this disease. It is in
malarious and neurotic cases especially, that arsenic is of
service.

Sub-acute eczema, affecting a considerable portion of
the body, will not yield to alkalies alone, and often seems
to depend entirely upon great general debility. It is then
necessary to give the most powerfully tonic treatment, at
the same time that great care is paid to the emunctories;
much may also be accomplished by baths, as described
elsewhere, together with proper local applications subsequently.

Chronic eczema may require the most varied and carefully regulated treatment, according to the conditions existing in each case. In other chapters it has been shown
that most eczema patients exhibit either assimilative,
nutritive, or nervous debility, and thought should be di-

rected to rectifying this gouty, strumous, or neurotic state present, as the first step in treatment.

I am aware that it may be claimed that much of what has been said in regard to the constitutional relations of eczema and what may follow in reference to their management, pertains as well to other diseases, and to persons exhibiting no eczema at all ; and also that many of the directions for treatment relate quite as much to those who would regain perfect health as to those affected with eczema. But in answer I would say that the present is a practical clinical study of the disease, and that the desire is simply to present the subject as it has developed itself in practice. Of the importance and necessity of attending to the matters here detailed in order to secure the best success, there is not a shadow of doubt in my mind, the features developed could each be demonstrated by hundreds of cases.

We are not, moreover, to consider these general matters in too general a manner, but must regard each of them as of real importance in the management of eczema ; for experience has abundantly shown that as the elements of these states remain active, the skin difficulty will tend to return again and again, if indeed it yields at all well to local treatment. And it must not be forgotten that the signs of systemic disease must generally be sought for or they will escape notice ; the interest of the patient is often so absorbed in the local lesion on the skin, that it is difficult to induce one to give attention to anything else. Multitudes go through life in a chronic condition of ill health, and never recognize it or give it thought, until some special disease attracts attention to their personal condition. Many, of course, accept this " below par " state, as their normal one, but when careful, thorough, and systematic treatment has been instituted and carried out for an eczema, it is continually found that the general health is better than for many years. In previous chapters, constipation, dyspepsia, and urinary disorders were stated to be very frequent accompaniments of eczema, and as evidences of faulty assimilation and disintegration these should receive most careful attention.

In regard to the constipation of eczema, it is not enough that casual inquiry be made as to the action of the bowels, and that general directions be given that the patient see to it that they are free; but the matter must be carefully inquired into, not only on the first visit, but also on each subsequent occasion. I am confident that in an imperfect secretion and excretion from the chylopoëtic viscera lies the cause not only of much eczema, but also of some other affections, both of the skin and other organs.

Quite recently serious attention has been directed by several writers to the importance of deranged liver action as a cause of uterine difficulty; and even of displacements and tumors. This I have long recognized from a medical standpoint, and have seen many cases presenting marked indications of uterine disease and ovarian irritation. and even some cases which had been treated unsuccessfully by gynæcologists, recover completely, and alone, under treatment instituted for a skin difficulty, often an eczema, where of necessity much attention was paid to the liver and bowel condition.

In many instances the action of the bowels is irregular or defective from neglect, and if the importance of securing a free movement every morning, directly after breakfast, is appreciated by the patient, and acted upon, much less medication will be necessary ; this early evacuation of the bowels is often neglected by school children and business men, also greatly by women. Neglect to empty the rectum favors absorption of the liquid portion of the fæces, and the stools are hard, dark, and lumpy. I believe that an imperfect emptying of the bowels may often result from the withdrawal of nerve influence, and I therefore discountenance the practice, common with many, of reading the newspaper while at stool ; we know well how nervous excitement may cause the imperative desire to evacuate the rectum, and nervous suspense or activity may in a similar manner lead to the retention of fæcal matter. I have also reason to believe that smoking at stool renders the evacuation less perfect.

The very common practice of securing a discharge from the bowels by means of enemata is not to be commended, certainly not in the management of eczema. This is but a local process, stimulating the sluggish rectum to eject its contents, while it has the further disadvantage of supplying the fluid which should be furnished by the intestine itself. This does not assist in removing the effete products of disassimilation from the economy, it does not excite the action of the liver or upper bowel, but is only a scavenging process for conveying away that which has been already collected ; it actually does harm both by covering up a failure in the action of other organs, and by taking away the stimulus afforded by a full rectum. I find this practice of relying upon enemata a very common one in eczema patients, and always seek to supplant it by securing a healthy alvine evacuation. I believe the cases are exceedingly rare where, if a proper intestinal excretion is presented to the rectum that organ will be incapable of expelling it. When there seems to be simply atony of the lower bowel, nux vomica pushed almost to tolerance will be of the greatest service, as I have repeatedly seen. The necessity of using enemata results very frequently from carelessness, either from the frequent neglect to heed the call of nature, or from the ignorant continuance of a habit first practiced to relieve a slight constipation from some transient cause.

Nor is it better to pour the water into the other end of the intestinal tube, as is constantly done with the laxa-

tive mineral waters, which latter have undoubtedly been
productive of much evil from their constant abuse. If digestion proceeds properly and if sufficient exercise is taken,
the intestine will not require such stimulation. I am confident that while both enemata and mineral waters are
frequently taken with the idea of obviating the evil results
of the intestinal inactivity resulting from sedentary habits,
over-indulgence at the table, etc., they in reality do harm
by hurrying on the bowel action, and making a show of
securing complete evacuations, while the real source of
evil is left untouched.

It does not answer, therefore, simply to direct that the
patient with eczema keep the bowels open with one or the
other of the mineral waters ; I see many patients who have
followed this advice from others, whose constipation practically remained and whose eczema had still persisted most
rebelliously ; I very rarely order the mineral waters for this
purpose, and constantly stop their use. Constipation is
frequently only a sign of debility, and the tonic treatment
to be described, together with the dietetic and hygienic
measures of service in the management of the eczema will
often be the means of establishing a regularity in this function even in those in whom it has been long deranged. The
abuse of purgatives is undoubtedly a very frequent cause
of constipation, and great care and patience may be required to bring patients out from their continued dependence upon intestinal stimulants ; but this can and should
be accomplished even at considerable pains.

In regard to the actual medical treatment of the element of constipation in eczema, it is well to ensure free
action from the bowels at the commencement of the treatment, especially before giving a tonic course of iron, etc.,
and this should be repeated from time to time if there is
sluggishness of action, or if the breath becomes foul or the
tongue coated. It is particularly desirable to attend to

this during the administration of arsenic. As a thorough and safe laxative under these circumstances nothing answers better than the pills before alluded to, of blue mass, colocynth and ipecac (Formula 13), or the Pilula Cambogiæ Composita is a good substitute. For overcoming habitual constipation the pills of aloes and iron (Formula 14), used in diminishing numbers as described in the chapter on eczema of the anus and genital region, will be found most effective. Further reference to this subject will be made in connection with eczema of various regions of the body.

The management of the dyspepsia or imperfect digestion accompanying eczema will occasionally give the greatest trouble, and in some cases almost every available method of treatment may be resorted to before complete relief is obtained. No precise rules or indications for treatment can be given in this general consideration of the subject, so different are the cases ; suffice it to state that careful attention must be paid to every particular, the diet being also regulated with the utmost care, not only with reference to the good or bad effect of articles of diet upon the eczema, but especially in regard to their action upon the digestive organs. As to medication, in one case alkalies are required, in another the mineral acids, and in a third pepsin or some pure bitter ; often many of them combined. Placing this feature of the case on a health footing is the first step towards the cure of the eczema.

Urinary derangements were shown to be frequent, and present indications which should always be considered and acted upon in accordance with the rules of general medicine.

When the strumous state is found to exist, cod-liver oil, syrup of the lacto-phosphate of lime, syrup of the phosphates of lime, soda, and iron, iodide of iron, etc., are of inestimable value, together with extra nourishment, especially in the line of fats. But here it must never be forgotten that there may be, and often is, assimilative disorder as well in strumous subjects, which requires treatment before the nutritive measures can act.

Patients exhibiting the nervous state may also require much attention in the matter of the digestive functions, which are often greatly impaired ; not at all infrequently what appears to be a neurasthenic case, will be found to owe its neurotic symptoms almost, if not quite entirely to imperfect digestion. But many cases, again, exhibit most marked and clear nervous elements, which require special attention and treatment. Nerve tonics, strychnine, quinine, the preparations of phosphorus and arsenic, with also cod-liver oil, iron, etc., perhaps with the addition of electricity, may be required to cure the eczema, and under their use comes also an improvement of the other general symptoms. Often, however, rest, change of scene and travel alone are of benefit, and the eruption will resist all treatment until these are added.

Arsenic and its preparations have long been held in high repute in the treatment of eczema, as well as of other affections of the skin ; and its reputation is undoubtedly well founded, both upon the physiological effects of the drug, and upon the results often obtained in practice. It certainly does often seem to control eczema better than any other single remedy, when given in sufficient quantities, especially in children, as I have shown elsewhere.*
But as may be judged from what has been stated of the nature and causes of eczema, arsenic is by no means indicated in every case ; it was probably not given at all in one half of the cases here analyzed. As a modifier of cutaneous nutrition, it is often of value in chronic cases, but used alone and indiscriminately, it may often do harm. It is especially indicated in nervous cases, and those exhibit-

---

* The use and value of Arsenic in the treatment of Diseases of the Skin. New York Medical Journal, August, 1876.

ing a malarious element. I do not know of any very essential difference in the action of the various preparations of arsenic, but not at all infrequently one combination will be tolerated and be of service, when another irritates.

Mercury in minute doses is sometimes of great service as an alterative in chronic eczema, not only in cases presenting an old syphilitic history, but also in those where this is not even suspected.

Iodide of potassium is seldom of value and often very harmful in eczema, and is rarely called for. Donovan's solution presents no advantages over extemporaneous prescriptions made when arsenic, mercury, and iodine are called for; it is very seldom employed by those who see much of eczema.

The itching of eczema is often so troublesome a feature that the patient will cry loudly for relief from this symptom, and the thoughts of the physician will often be turned away from the real and proper treatment of the disease in his attempts to allay the distress and to quiet the clamor of the sufferer. It must always be borne in mind that the quickest and surest help is to be found in the correct treatment of the case in question, and that efforts to give much or permanent relief while the cruption exists will generally result in failure, and often in harm to the eruption. Caution must therefore be exercised in resorting to local applications for this purpose, for one not infrequently sees eczema greatly irritated by the stronger and stronger applications which have been made in the attempt to alleviate the itching.

Nor can so very much be done directly by internal remedies to ease the itching, and the list of medicines which have a definite action in this direction is very small. Morphia and opium are not infrequently prescribed in the hope of giving relief, but they are if anything worse than useless, often increasing the pruritus; and if by their

means the patient gets sleep, it is unrefreshing and disturbed by tormenting dreams, during which the sufferer
is working at the affected parts. Belladonna given internally is said to give some relief, but only in full doses,
which may prove dangerous. Carbolic acid has been
given internally with some results in prurigo, but it does
not seem to alleviate the itching of eczema when taken.
Chloral and bromide of potassium alone or combined are
often of the greatest service for temporary relief, but
should be used cautiously, as their depressant action
harms the eczema in the end; aconite may be added to
them with good effect at times.

During the past few years I have been employing
gelsemium for this purpose with good results in selected
cases, and reported favorably upon it in a recent number
of the New York Medical Journal, January, 1881. It is,
of course, not always successful, but as an adjuvant it
often serves a very good end. The tincture was used exclusively in my cases, and given at first in ten drop doses,
repeated and increased every half hour until the patient
was relieved or experienced physiological symptoms.
The effects of the drug are a sense of languor and
tranquillity, slight dizziness, impairment of vision, and
drooping of the lids; later a feeling of numbness and
embarrassment of the heart's action, and enfeebled respiration, and even vertigo and ptosis may come on from
an over dose. I have never seen any unpleasant
effects, but have never had the medicine pushed much,
seldom allowing much more than a drachm to be taken
in all within two hours; but it should be stated that in
very rare cases even a smaller dose than that mentioned,
a few drops, has been followed by alarming symptoms, but
no evil results, as far as I can discover, have been reported from medicinal doses. I have generally given it at
bedtime, and a single dose or two has often afforded much

relief. In some cases I have prescribed it in repeated doses during the day with decided effect. I have never given it to children.

To return to the subject of the constitutional treatment of eczema. Suppose a case does not apparently present the features described, and there seem to be no indications for internal treatment, the patient claiming to be, and apparently being in perfect health with the single exception of the eruption which is presented for treatment : what is to be done in such a case ? It may be answered that very careful investigation will generally detect the conditions which have been described, and will mark out a line of management, for true eczema is not a purely local affection of the skin. If, however, no sufficient reasons for a general constitutional course of management are discovered, two lines of treatment still remain to be followed. First, believing eczema to be a disease of debility, primarily constitutional, with a subsequent sharing of the local tissues in the general lowered vitality, we may prescribe a tonic course of regimen and diet, with tonics such as iron, bark, etc. ; quinine is added if in a malarious subject or locality, or arsenic, with perhaps an alkali, or an acid, care being taken during the treatment that the emunctories act freely : or, second, upon the supposition that a transient systemic cause may have passed away, and with a view of removing the local debility and the infiltration or the *products* of the disease, special attention is given to local treatment alone.

This introduces that portion of the subject of the management of eczema which usually gives the practitioner the most difficulty, and in which perhaps the greatest numbers of errors are made, namely, the proper applications to be made to parts affected with eczema. As in the consideration of the general therapeutics special remedies were left to be detailed in subsequent chapters, so the special local applications suitable to particular parts and conditions will be more particularly dwelt on later in connection with eczema of the various regions. There are, however, some general considerations which are of the highest importance, which may be best treated of in this place.

The first point to be considered in determining upon a suitable local application is, in regard to the stage of the eruption, that is the acute, sub-acute, or chronic character of the lesions to be treated, for the measures which are applicable to the one are often entirely unsuited to the other: the applications which are of value in acute eczema are powerless in the chronic forms, while those which are serviceable in the chronic states may be and generally are highly injurious to the inflammatory condition of acute eczema.

By far the greatest number of errors, which are distressing to the patient and annoying to the physician, are in the direction of too stimulating or too irritating applications, and the great lesson to learn is the intense irritability of the skin in acute and often in sub-acute eczema. A soothing plan of treatment must be adopted in the earlier stages of the disease: it is far better to err by not doing enough than it is to over stimulate a part already suffering from the effects of irritation.

The principles of local treatment, therefore, are essentially, to soothe and moderate, or modify inflammatory action in the early, acute, or sub-acute stages by emollients, protectives and mild astringents, and to stimulate or excite healthy absorptive action in the later or chronic stages, phases, or conditions of the disease. The physician therefore must determine in regard as to the condition present in each case and the measures suited to it, and not employ any one remedy for all stages, nor any particular application because reported as valuable in eczema, upon however high an authority. In other words the physician must definitely know and appreciate for what conditions any particular treatment is recommended, and also know and appreciate the state of the parts to be treated in the particular case under consideration; he should also understand the action of the remedies to be used, and then apply them according to the principles here laid down.

This will assuredly require some thought, and even with the best instructions some experience is necessary in order to form a correct judgment in this as in every other line of medical practice. I will now attempt to indicate more particularly the items worthy of special consideration. ·

First, it should be well borne in mind in managing every case of eczema that both air and water are irritants to the surface bared of its normal epidermis by the disease; nature seeks continually to cover the exposed tissues, but the formation is imperfect, the epidermal cells are cast off with the serous exudation, they form scales and crusts of varying thickness, but with no cohesion, with no adaptability to the protection of the part. If now, this process is allowed to go on, it repeats itself almost indefinitely and we constantly see eczematous surfaces which have exuded for months or years with little or no tendency to spontaneous cure. Protection with soothing and astringent remedies therefore is necessary to allow the irritated cells of the part to undergo their proper transformation and hardening, and to protect the soft tissues beneath, and to allay capillary and nerve excitement.

It may be understood, therefore, how much harm may come from the indiscriminate and improper use of soap in eczema, and the very great injury which is done by such as are advertised to cure all eruptions, as sulphur and tar soaps, cuticura soap, carbolic soap, or even the various so-called soothing soaps; if applied to an acute eruption they but irritate an abraded surface, if used injudiciously in a chronic state, and without proper subsequent protection, the diseased part is excited to renewed activity, but the process of repair is not allowed to take place in a proper manner.

Soap frequently does play an important part in the treatment of eczema, but to be beneficial it must be of the right kind and properly employed, as will be detailed in connection with the management of the eruption in different localities. In general, however, it may be stated that washing with soap, as ordinarily understood, is prejudicial to eczema, and no advertised healing qualities can obviate the bad effects which follow. In persons with a tendency to eczema, some care must be exercised in reference to the soap commonly used, for many are either too alkaline or contain elements, as coloring matter, etc., which render them harmful. The safest soap in general, is old white Castile soap; Pear's English transparent soap is perhaps as good as can be found. Sulphur and tar soaps are generally too stimulating for constant use. Eczematous subjects should be careful to dry the skin perfectly after washing, and the subsequent use of a glycerine lotion (Formula 37), or a glycerite of starch ointment (Formula 73), will prevent further trouble.

In regard to the applications of service in eczema, it must be premised that a certain amount of uncertainty attends the action of all local remedies, on account of individual differences in the skin of different patients, so that sometimes a measure which has proved of service in what appears to be quite a similar case, will aggravate instead of benefiting an eruption. It may also be stated that it is not always as important as to what remedy is used, as it is in what manner it is employed; that is, there are many remedies which have a similar action, and they may often be prescribed indifferently, provided the desired aim, protection and an astringent action is secured. This is often demonstrated in a public clinic, where a series of similar cases will each receive a different treatment with equal success.

To protect and soothe acute eczematous surfaces, three kinds or varieties of applications may be used ; dusting powders, lotions, and ointments. In an acutely inflamed eczema, with the development of vesicles or pustules, with much burning heat, a dusting powder is the most suitable application. For this purpose simple rice powder, or fine buckwheat flour, or powdered starch answer very well, also lycopodium, talc or French chalk, and carbonate of magnesium. These may also be variously combined with astringents, and with camphor or a little morphine if there is burning heat or tingling, in the manner described in other chapters (Formulæ 23, 24, 25, 26).

Moist applications are also often of very great service in the acute stages of eczema, and those combinations are preferable, which on drying leave a powdery deposit on the surface (Formulæ 31, 32, 33, 34, 35). Such lotions yield their results in part by their evaporation, and, therefore, should not be used with thick folds of linen, nor be kept covered with impermeable dressing, as oiled-silk, for the application is then converted into a poultice, and the parts are soddened and weakened, instead of being astringed and strengthened. But the powder of these lotions should not be allowed to dry on too greatly, and form too much of a coating over the parts, because decomposing secretions may thus be retained, and a dry, hard crust may be formed which is irritating instead of soothing. The parts, therefore, may require occasional gentle bathing with tepid water, made mildly alkaline by bi-carbonate of soda or borax, a teaspoonful or so to the pint ; or with bran water or oatmeal water, or, I not infrequently direct that some of the alkaline bath water, containing starch, as described elsewhere, be kept and used occasionally for washing. The powder or lotion is to be immediately reapplied after washing, to protect the parts from the air. In many cases no better local application can be made, than a lead and opium wash (Formula 39), or the black wash of the pharmacopœia, bathed on the part, or applied on muslin ; it is generally better to use an ointment at night, as one with a very little zinc, for as the wash is apt to dry and adhere to the diseased surface, violence may be done when the cloth is torn off.

Most of the lotions above alluded to are made with a little glycerine, which greatly facilitates the adhering of the powder which they contain, and keeps the parts supple. It must ever be borne in mind that some skins will not bear glycerine, even greatly diluted ; in these cases another demulcent may be substituted, such as the almond emulsion, or decoction of marshmallow.

I may here make a remark in regard to the method of making applications ; a sponge should never be used in connection with the treatment of skin diseases ; not only is it dirty, and may become the means of spreading contagious diseases, but it is irritating to the skin, and absorbs the fluid of an application, leaving any powder held in solution clinging to it, and the pressure used to expel the liquid may be more than is desirable. Soft old linen cloths should be employed ; or when ointments are to be applied the surgeon's lint is preferable. When stimulation is desired, as will be mentioned later, white flannel may be used with advantage.

As a rule, ointments and all greasy applications are not well borne in acutely inflamed eczema, and must be applied with caution ; if they are used they should not be rubbed on the surface but spread upon muslin or lint, and laid carefully on the part, care being taken to change the dressing with as little irritation as possible, two or more times daily; the secretion must not be confined, as it may prove very irritating to adjacent parts. None but the most soothing ointments must be used, such as oxide or carbonate of zinc, half a drachm to the ounce of rose ointment, or bismuth sub-nitrate in the same proportions. I have found cucumber ointment even more soothing than the rose ointment to an acutely inflamed skin. The preparations of petroleum, vaseline and cosmoline, are not as serviceable for ointments as it was hoped they would prove; owing to their great fluidity at the temperature of the body, they do not hold the medicament in position, nor protect the parts from the air sufficiently well. Their freedom from rancidity is a very strong recommendation, for fatty matter which is at all rancid is most irritating to the skin. The glycerite of starch is often most valuable as an excipient in ointments.

No allusion has been made to the use of poultices in acute eczema, for the reason that although they are not infrequently advised in general practice they are not of real service in treating this disease, and are rarely used in the practice of Dermatology. As a very rare application to soften a hard surface or to remove crust they may sometimes be of service, but the maceration of a poultice weakens the tissues too much, and in the end harm is apt to be done.

The local treatment of chronic eczema is quite another affair. In acute eczema we have a more or less self-limited, congestive eruption, and the object of treatment is to carry it through its stages as quickly as possible; to this end we seek to moderate inflammatory action by removing external irritants and protecting the surface by soothing and slightly astringent applications, and thus, while hastening the process we aim to prevent the infiltration of the skin.

Chronic eczema on the other hand represents more the product of the disease, the infiltration, together with a chronic dilatation of the blood-vessels and lymphatics of the part: against these such mild, local measures as have been mentioned are almost powerless, and recourse must be had to stimulation, combined with measures which limit the action of the stimulant, and induce absorption.

Hebra, observing that when there is free secretion from the surface the itching of eczema is much diminished, made a bold dash in the way of local therapeutics and demonstrated the curability by a stimulating treatment, of many cases of chronic eczema which were otherwise and previously quite if not wholly incurable. This plan consists in the application of such agents and in such a manner as will remove at once and entirely the imperfectly formed epithelial layers (which would be thrown off sooner or later), thus giving vent to the pent-up exudation, and stimulating the skin so violently as really to induce an acute eruption. For this purpose he directs that patches of chronic eczema shall be scrubbed energetically with soft, potassa soap, by means of flannel or stiff brushes, to such a degree as even to cause the foam produced by the addition of water to be red with blood, as I have repeatedly witnessed; and upon this raw surface thus occasioned cold and wet compresses are laid and frequently changed, or the diachylon ointment, spread upon linen; the stimulating process is repeated once or twice during twenty-four hours. In certain cases of thickened eczema, as on the scrotum, Hebra also applies a poultice of the same green soap, with the effect of completely dissolving and removing the outer layers of the skin and producing a free exudation from the surface. He further advises very strong solutions of caustic potassa, even up to equal parts with water by weight, to be well rubbed on infiltrated patches, certainly to the great relief of the itching and removal of the infiltration, as I have observed frequently.

But my experience is that American skins will not always stand these very harsh applications ; nor will our patients always submit to such painful treatment, requiring ofttimes confinement to the bed and generally a cessation of occupation, for diseases which affect their comfort and pleasure mainly, and do not endanger life ; and further, I find that the same ends may generally be accomplished by other and milder means.

These very severe remedies, moreover, cannot always be employed with impunity, even by Hebra himself. I perfectly recall an occurrence in his out-patient clinic, where a young girl about eighteen years of age applied for the treatment of a small patch of sub-acute eczema on the back of one of her hands. Hebra had just been manipulating another patient with a very strong solution of potassa, and he rubbed the swab in his hand over the patch, intimating as she left that it might cause trouble if it did not cure. In a few days the patient presented herself for admission to the hospital, with the whole hand swollen and painful ; the entire arm was soon involved in a very severe suppurative eczema, which spread somewhat on the body, and was accompanied with a very high fever. She was in the hospital some time and suffered much, and all this from the injudicious use of a caustic, and that in the hands of Hebra. Surely others have need of caution.

Great thanks are, however, due to the German school for the development of local pathology, and the local treatment of many diseases of the skin, and especially for the introduction of the use of stimulants and tarry applications in chronic eczema ; when judiciously employed, these are of great service in relieving the itching and reducing the infiltration of the skin accompanying this disease.

While the more severe degrees of local stimulating treatment are not always well borne, still in a modified form the plans advocated by Hebra are of great value and are often called for in rebellious cases; especially are they of service where single, isolated patches of hard, chronic eczema linger long in spite of other and well directed internal and local management. This harsh treatment should never be applied to very large or numerous surfaces. In order to properly appreciate and understand this plan of treatment, to the end that it may be carried out to the letter, it is to be remembered that the object of the treatment is to remove the imperfectly formed outer layers of cuticle, and to induce healthy action in the cells of the skin. I will briefly describe the way in which this may be accomplished, following as far as possible the account given by Professor Hebra.

A portion of the potash soap, sapo viridis (or green soap) the size of a walnut is spread upon a bit of flannel and rubbed with firm pressure upon the eczematous patch for several minutes, the flannel being occasionally dipped in water in order to form a lather upon the part. After the operation has lasted several minutes, according to the effect, the surface is washed free from the soap and the suitable ointment, generally the diachylon (Formula 61), is applied, it having been previously spread thickly on the wooly side of a piece of lint large enough to wholly cover the diseased part.

The frictions with soap are repeated morning and evening with such force and for such a length of time, that small excoriated points are seen upon the eczematous patch. It should be mentioned that moderate friction with this green soap produces no morbid appearances upon the healthy skin, but after being washed off the surface is left smooth and feeling agreeably. In contrast to the effect upon the healthy skin are the appearances presented by an eczematous patch thus treated, which shows numerous, intensely red, moist points bereft of epidermis, caused by the destruction, by means of the soap, of the epidermal layers which had been undermined by the eczema fluid and had formed the vesicles. While after the first frictions a large number of these red, moist, shiny points are seen, and to the unpracticed eye the eczema appears to be worse, these points grow smaller after subsequent frictions, until finally they entirely disappear, and the previously diseased surface assumes the character of the healthy tissue and is no longer affected by the soap. In small, very chronic patches of eczema, frictions with solutions of caustic potash may sometimes be used with excellent results, as will be mentioned elsewhere.

The details of the local treatment of eczema, must be reserved for particular description in connection with the various manifestations of the disease in different localities, for these are so varied that no general directions can be given with profit. The main principle to be borne in mind, however, is that if stimulant measures are adopted, they should be brisk and sharp, and time should be given for a reaction to take place. Prolonged, or too frequent, or inefficient stimulation may be harmful, it being only another form of *irritation*, such as the tissue had been previously subjected to, with an aggravation of the lesion ; whereas, short, active, energetic stimulation, such even as that given by cantharides, followed by a proper reaction, results in restored activity to the circulation and absorption of the exuded product, or infiltration.

CHAPTER IX.

THE MANAGEMENT OF INFANTILE ECZEMA.

THE term infantile eczema is here applied to those cases of this disease occurring in children five years of age or under, although writers have not generally been very definite in fixing upon the time of life at which it ceases to be properly so called. The reasons for making a separate class of all cases of eczema developed during this period are found not so much in any essential peculiarities in the disease, as in certain characteristics which the eruption presents, certain causes which occasion it, and certain methods of procedure in its management. The disease which begins during the earliest months of existence may last many years, even to full adult life, or indefinitely. But the age of five years is chosen as the point at which the eruption ceases to be regarded as infantile eczema because at this period there is a very considerable diminution in the number of newly developed cases, owing to the cessation of many of the causes which had previously operated.

The periods of life are conveniently divided into decades and half decades, and if we look at the statistics of a large number of cases of eczema, we find that the first ten years of life present a very much greater proportion of cases than any other equal period; and nearly three-fourths of the cases occurring during this decade, will be found in children five years or less of age. Thus of the three thousand cases of eczema here analyzed, 907, or almost one-third, occurred during the first ten years of life, and of these, 676 were observed in children five years old or under ; that is, almost twenty-five per cent. or nearly one-quarter of the entire number of cases of eczema came within the definition of infantile eczema. It would seem that infantile eczema is more common in this country than in England ; Mr. Wilson states the proportion of infantile to other cases of eczema at one to sixteen, or only a little over six per cent. I cannot otherwise understand his statistics, for his limits of age must be about the same as are here given, inasmuch as he speaks of a number of the cases having lasted from six months to four years and a half, at the time of consultation.

This proportion which I have recorded, would undoubtedly be increased very largely, if all the cases of eczema occurring in a community were collected, or even if the cases coming under the care of family physicians were tabulated, instead of those taken from a consulting practice, where, in the main, the more obstinate and severe cases only are met with, and a very considerable number of mild cases escape observation and record. Also in the statistics taken from public practice, there is a smaller number of cases of infantile eczema than there should be, owing to the fact that in public institutions, many children with skin diseases find their way to the children's department, and are consequently not entered upon the books from which these statistics are gathered.

Undoubtedly also in both classes of practice, multitudes of cases are never treated at all, owing to the impression so prevalent among the laity and the profession, that it is dangerous or useless to treat this disorder. The layman fears lest some harm may come from the disease being " driven in," which fear the physician sometimes unconsciously fosters from ignorance, or oftener from carelessness and unwillingness to cope with the case.

The little sufferer from eczema, therefore, is left to bear his trials unaided, under the hope that with each change in its physiological conditions the disease will pass away. Thus, the eruption being called "milk crust" during nursing, the assurance is given that it will cease when it cuts its teeth. When this stage is arrived at, and the condition is aggravated with each accession of a tooth, the eruption takes the name of " tooth-rash," and it is expected that it will cease when certain teeth are developed. These come and yet the disease proceeds, little being done to check or modify it, and so the eruption continues, and by the long duration of the disease and the causes which occasion it, the eczematous habit, diathesis, or condition is acquired, and the eruption may be prolonged in a chronic form perhaps during the entire life. I have seen multitudes of cases which had lasted not only many months, but even one, two, four or more years. Indeed I have seen a characteristic eczema, a veritable milk-crust, which had remained on the head from earliest infancy to twelve years of age. In another case a gentleman of thirty-one years of age had had the same on the legs since the first years of life ; and in still other instances the disease which had begun in earliest infancy, had lasted from twenty to fifty years.

It is by no means denied that attacks of eczema in infants are often intimately associated with a faulty milk diet, and with the development and cutting of teeth, but it is absolutely denied that eczema is a necessary result of either the partaking of milk or the irruption of teeth; and it can be shown beyond doubt that eczema always and invariably signifies an error of some kind which medical thought should avert ; and that it is, like any other aberration from health, a condition of affairs which medical skill should remove.

It may also be very clearly and definitely stated, that

there is and can be absolutely no harm resulting from curing eczema in infants any more than in adults. This statement is made not only from long experience with the disease, but with a knowledge of the opinions of others who are accounted able to judge in this matter; although it is true that older writers have sometimes stated to the contrary. It has already been shown in the preceding chapters, that eczema is not the result of an internal ferment or poison seeking exit from the system, and that the lesion upon the skin is not beneficial in any sense of the word. The eruption is the result of altered nutrition and assimilation, and that these are relieved or the patient benefited by the exudation or by the continuance of the eczema, is absolutely denied. Consequently there is not the slightest danger of the eruption either "striking in" or of its being "driven in"; there is no danger that "the disease" may fly to some other part if the disorder on the skin is removed.

Nor is it true that convulsions or an internal disease can result from the cure of an eczema; in not one instance of the more than six hundred cases of infantile eczema here analyzed have any such results ever occurred. Nor have I ever had occasion to regret successful treatment. But on the other hand, exactly the contrary result has happened; namely, that former sufferers from eczema have gained in health and strength after the removal of their exhausting skin difficulty.

It is true indeed, that patients with eczema do acquire other diseases occasionally in the course of treatment, quite as often as though they were not suffering with eczema. It is also true that, in some instances, an internal inflammation may result from a chilling of the surface during exposure in baths or otherwise, in connection with the treatment of eczema. But all recent authorities are entirely agreed in this matter, that such disorders are not due to the skin disease " striking in," indeed that they have no connection with the eruption, and that the coincidence is accidental. On the other hand it can be shown, that if internal disease, as a fever, attacks a person with a cutaneous affection who is not under treatment, the skin disorder may disappear for awhile, only to return when the internal or general sickness ceases. But it cannot be shown that the curing of an external disease has ever resulted in one affecting any other organ of the body. A striking confirmation of this is found in Vienna, where the treatment of skin diseases is almost entirely by means of local remedies, and those who know most about it, insist positively that no harm has ever come within their experience from the proper treatment of the cutaneous disease, even by external measures.

Infantile eczema presents certain features different from the phases of the disorder which are ordinarily seen in adult life ; and these appear to be largely dependent upon the structure and quality of the skin of children. After its prolonged intra-uterine maceration it is exceedingly delicate and soft at birth, and is by no means as hard and tough as it becomes in after life. Even during the first months or years of life the skin is still tender and sensitive, and hardly able to withstand the comparatively rough treatment of the external world, and the irritating agencies to which it is constantly exposed. Causes which in later life may be entirely inoperative, here induce congestion and inflammation with the greatest ease, while the many other disturbing influences of heat and cold, improper food, and nervous excitement, continually tend to derange the equilibrium of the forces which seek to form a perfect frame. The frequency of eczema in childhood is but a part of the frequency of all other diseases, with the added local causes of the exposure to constant outward irritation, of a most delicate and complex structure.

The expression, "the management of infantile ecze-ma" is peculiarly appropriate, because of the protean appearances which the disease presents, together with the greatly varied etiological factors and the many elements to be considered in connection with it. The measures to be employed in its cure are, therefore, to be considered in the light of a management of the patient, in all the relations of life, rather than as a definite treatment to be given, simply because the eruption of eczema is present.

It is impossible to describe fully and minutely all the phases which may appear in infantile eczema. They are simply those belonging to the disease itself in all its stages and conditions, as are described in other chapters.

When most severe the eruption may occupy all or a greater portion of the body, but this is comparatively rare, and in by far the larger proportion of the cases we have the eruption most developed and most marked about the face and head. The cheeks are perhaps more frequently first affected than any other portion, and here it often lingers long after it has disappeared from every other part of the body. The eruption usually begins as a reddened patch of varying size, generally exhibiting papules : this is itchy and is torn and rubbed, and the affected area may increase with great rapidity, a serous exudation being poured out which dries into crusts and scales, to be again torn off in the attempts to get relief from the itching.

It is not uncommon to have almost the entire head and face the seat of an acutely developed infantile cc-zema, which will vary in intensity from time to time. This is what is commonly called the crusta lactea, or milk crust, and according to the case, may either present a reddened and moist, or a moderately scaly and very itchy surface; or, crusts of considerable thickness may form, which, particularly upon the scalp, have a yellowish, gummy appearance, beneath which the surface is found to be still raw and exuding. The itching endured by the little sufferers when the disease is at all severe, is something terrible to witness. They continually seek to tear and rub the surface, and when prevented from so doing, will cry in agony. Nor does night afford any relief, and the watching parents will continually state that night after night for weeks or months, the infant has had almost no rest, only falling off into a doze from time to time, to awaken in a few moments, tearing its surface. If the child is prevented by physical restraint from scratching or rubbing with the hands, it will seek in some other way to allay the intolerable distress of the itching, by friction against the pillow, or against the shoulder of its attendant or its own shoulder.

Closely allied to or associated with eczema in infants and small children, is the formation of cutaneous abscesses, especially about the scalp. These may be so large and numerous, that a great portion of the head may be covered, either at once or by their successive development. They appear as masses of purplish red color, of various sizes and shapes, in which fluctuation may soon be detected; the inflammation is generally of a low grade, there is not nearly the pain connected with them which would be expected, and when they have attained some size, the skin over them becomes much thinned, and they readily break or are opened with comparatively little pain, and shrink down and heal very quickly. The pus is found to be of a poor, grumous quality, often dark and mixed with blood. These abscesses are found in exhausted children, generally of a strumous habit, and are especially common in summer. They yield easily, as a rule, to the treatment of eczema, described later, but they are particularly controlled by the sulphide of calcium in doses of about one tenth to one sixth of a grain, four or five times daily on an empty stomach.

The ears will frequently be involved in the process of eczema, and are then red, moist, and swollen. Sometimes they will be affected alone or together with the cheeks, or with other parts ; or there may be only a moderately moist, red surface of varying extent behind one or both of them, with fissures at the junction of the ear and scalp. The eyelids are often attacked during the later years of this period, and their edges become thickened and red, with crusts attached to the cilia, and in the morning the exudation may glue the eyelids together. The nose itself is very frequently spared from eruption externally, but within we may have crusts, which almost block up the nostril.

In milder cases, or after the severity of the disease has passed, the eruption takes the form of diffused, reddened, and slightly thickened patches, more or less scaly on the surface, and frequently exhibiting greater or less papulation ; this is also accompanied often by very severe itching. In infantile eczema of the trunk and extremities especially, there is commonly a certain amount of papulation, and the eruption is apt to take the form of patches of reddened and infiltrated tissue, of variable extent and shape, composed of aggregated papules which generally show signs of having been scratched, and present a certain amount of dried exudate on their surface.

In the flexures of the joints and in various places where the skin lies more or less in folds touching one another, as about the neck of fat infants, on the abdomen, groins, and nates, we more commonly have an evenly red surface, generally moist, constituting what is known as intertrigo, or better as eczema intertrigo. Scales or crusts are seldom seen here, but in places where the two surfaces of skin have been kept in close contact, we find a soft creamy or cheesy mass, composed of exfoliated epithelial cells and inflammatory exudation, often mingled with some powder which has been applied to heal the part. These raw, red, and moist patches come, and often go, very quickly, and a part which is apparently healthy one day, will on the next day present this appearance ; it is also astonishing how very rapidly the diseased portions will return again to the normal state under exactly proper treatment. These surfaces which seem so raw do not, as a rule, occasion much distress from itching, but sometimes the pain from them, especially when occurring about the groin and buttocks, may be very severe. The surface is raw and bereft of its natural epidermal covering, and the chafing of the clothing, or the irritation of cleansing may give much pain.

Eczema of the hands and arms in infants, and also of the feet and legs occasions much distress to the patient from the itching, and these parts are very frequently severely torn in scratching. Sometimes the eruption in the bends of the knees and elbows, especially during the later years of this period, is so severe, and accompanied by so much infiltration of tissue, that the parts crack and movement becomes very painful ; even to such a degree as to interfere with locomotion.

The diagnosis of. infantile eczema need not present great difficulties. There are but few conditions in children during this period, which can or should be confounded with the eruption here described. Sometimes the large, flat papules of inherited syphilis simulate eczema to a certain degree. But here the separate lesions can be made out with a little care, and the surface of the syphilitic eruption is of a much darker, coppery red, than that of eczema; the former is not attended with the thickening, itching, and moisture characteristic of eczema, and the scales if any are few, and quite firmly attached. The lesions of infantile syphilis are far more apt to be located, or to concentrate around the mouth and nose, also about the anus and genital region, and there can almost always be made out something of the circular or horse-shoe arrangement of the elements; at the corners of the mouth, the syphilitic eruption presents a certain pouting, which is characteristic, that is the papules or tubercles are a little elevated, soggy and very apt to present fissures. Around the anus and genital region the lesions are apt to be moist. Added to this, the presence of snuffles almost always found in syphilitic infants, the weasoned, old-man appearance of the face, and the syphilitic antecedents, and a picture is presented which should not be confounded with eczema.

Scabies in infants may resemble eczema to a certain degree, but in them, as in others, the eruption generally appears first upon the hands, especially between the fingers, and at the inner flexure of the wrist; likewise about the soles of the feet and ankles. The eruption is found to be multiform in scabies, that is, generally presenting papules, vesicles, and perhaps pustules, some of them of some size, while there are none of the even patches of exuding surface belonging to eczema. Furthermore it is rather easy in scabies upon children to discover the cuniculi or furrows made by the insect, as minute, brownish or black curved lines, looking as though a bit of dark sewing silk had been run beneath the skin, terminating at one extremity in a papule or pustule, or running over its surface. Very rarely if ever will infants with scabies present any lesions upon the face or scalp; if there is any general eruption at all it is papular, and the papules are separate and generally not a great deal scratched, as the itching is not as violent as in eczema. Contagion can almost invariably be made out in the case of infants with scabies.

Papular urticaria sometimes resembles eczema considerably. There is then a large portion of the surface of the body covered with scratched papules, more or less thickly set, and complaints are made of the restlessness of the child and its distress with itching.

But here we can always obtain the history of the acute and sudden development of the larger plaques or wheals belonging to urticaria, which disappear also rapidly, leaving the minute papule in the centre ; and generally the mark of the former wheal may be found as a slight, sharply defined erythematous blush, or halo around most of the papules.

Small infants are rarely if ever affected with the vegetable parasitic diseases, but during the later years of this period ringworm, and even favus are not so very uncommon. But here a careful examination will reveal their character, and the differential diagnosis may be made according to the rules pointed out in other chapters relating to eczema of various regions.

The prognosis of infantile eczema is invariably good, provided that all the elements of its management can be perfectly and properly carried out. Its cure is not only safe, but eminently proper and desirable. The duration of the treatment necessary can never be foretold exactly in any particular case ; it must vary greatly with the severity of the disease, the condition of the patient, the surroundings of the case, and the intelligence and obedience of the guardians. Mild cases may sometimes be entirely cured within a few days or weeks ; but in by far the larger proportion of instances, especially where the disease has already existed some time, the duration of the treatment must be counted by weeks or months. In severe cases the child should be watched by its medical attendant, and its mode of life superintended perhaps even for years, in order to prevent relapses.

The etiology of infantile eczema is most interesting and a subject worthy of the closest consideration, for upon its appreciation rests all true therapeutic success.

Sex appears to have but little influence in its production. Among our six hundred and seventy-six cases of infantile eczema there were three hundred and sixty-three males and three hundred and thirteen females ; in private practice the males presented yet a larger proportionate excess. In a few cases of infantile eczema analyzed by Mr. Wilson, the number of males was found to be nearly twice as great as that of females ; but he looked upon this as accidental, and I have not been able to discover any reason why male children should be more predisposed to this eruption than females.

Heredity has been shown in preceding chapters to be of little influence in the production of eczema. In but a small proportion of the cases met with were the parents, one or both, subjects of eczema, and conversely we continually see mothers and fathers with eczema, whose infants entirely escape. It is true, however, that many parents with a strong eczema tendency often do have children thus affected, although they themselves may not have any eruption at the particular time when the child happens to have it. But my studies have convinced me, upon close questioning of parents and others, from an investigation and discovery of other efficient causes, and from the results of treatment, that but little importance is to be attached to the element of heredity as an etiological factor in eczema of infants and children.

Eczema often appears to be contagious, especially among small children, as, when a whole family is said to be attacked, or when a nurse has it, after attending a child affected. But in these cases it is generally found that either the same influences are at work producing the disease in all the instances, or that some other eruption has been mistaken for that of eczema. Sometimes, however, we do see a small amount of transient local inflammation produced in another person from prolonged contact with the secretion, especially from a pustular eczema, and occasionally we find instances where the disease appears to be spread on a child, from the conveyance of the secretion from one portion to another. Here, however, we have to do simply with the irritating effects of animal secretions ; all pus is known to be more or less inoculable. But even in these cases real eczema is not produced, but simply a local dermatitis, which ends shortly when the local cause has ceased. Eczema as a disease, therefore, even in these cases, is not contagious.

We will first dismiss the subject of the local causes of infantile eczema, which can be done quite briefly. It has been claimed that the eruptive fevers are of etiological importance in this connection. But, as stated in a previous chapter, comparatively few children have eczema immediately after having undergone them, while a far larger number are affected with this eruption before they have passed through scarlet fever or measles ; and, further, I do not think it can be shown that any larger proportion of children who have had these diseases are affected with eczema, than of those who have not. My experience certainly entirely confirms this.

The opinion is very prevalent among the laity, and one hears it even in the profession, that vaccination has been the cause of the eczema, and in quite a share of the cases of this disease in children the charge is made that the child was vaccinated with "bad pock," and that the eruption resulted therefrom. Now it is true that in many instances the eruption will appear very shortly after the child has been vaccinated, either starting from the point of insertion of the virus or appearing elsewhere. But, many have eczema either before vaccination or long afterwards, and on the other hand, multitudes are vaccinated without ever having eczema, and I constantly vaccinate eczematous subjects, and even during the existence of an eruption, without ill effect. From what we know of the nature and constitutional relations of eczema, and of the nature and course of the vaccine disease, it may be positively asserted that vaccination cannot cause eczema, although like any other cutaneous irritant, it may provoke an eruption in one strongly inclined thereto.

Too frequent and too severe washing and cleansing of a part, is often an exciting cause of eczema in infants and very young children ; their tissues are not yet formed so as to resist the action of soaps, which are often too alkaline.

Eczema of the scalp is often started by the efforts put forth to remove the sebaceous collections which sometimes form here upon infants and children, and, from a very small spot of eczema thus begun, the skin irritation may proceed to the formation of large eczematous tracts.

Exposure to cold seems to be frequently an exciting cause of the appearance of eczema upon the face of infants ; and possibly the reason for the frequent occurrence of the eruption upon the scalp is found in the character of the very warm head-dressings used at one time, and the great exposure of the head to drafts at another. Irritating diapers are constantly found to be a source of eczema, and harsh cleansing of the lower parts also occasions it. On the other hand neglect of cleanliness of these regions, and the irritation of the excreta upon them will sometimes be found to excite the eruption.

The fact cannot be denied, that very many infants with eczema, perhaps the majority, look to be' in perfect health, indeed may be apparently healthier than others in the family who have not the eruption.   They are not infrequently of a ruddy color, have a good appetite, and are said to have regular action of the bowels, and parents are with difficulty convinced that there is any error beyond the simple skin lesion.   And yet I feel confident in affirming that exceedingly careful medical investigation will always discover something to be corrected besides the disorder of the skin; certain it is that a very rigid investigation and regulation of the diet, mode of life, etc., together with appropriate aid from medicines, accomplishes for these little ones what local treatment alone.has often failed to do.

The effect of the diet upon eczema in infants and small children, and the importance of giving the very strictest attention to it, can hardly be over-estimated. This subject will be very fully presented in the chapter on the diet and hygiene of eczema.

Constipation is a very frequent accompaniment of eczema in infants as well as adults, though the reverse state, diarrhœa, is occasionally met with.   Either and both are evidences of mal-assimilation.   In the beginning of the treatment, nothing that I know of suits so well to unload the bowels and make an impression on the eczema as calomel, in doses suited to the age and condition of the child. Under a year, I generally give a grain or a little less, rubbed up with sugar or with a little bi-carbonate of soda (Formula 19); the dose being increased about half a grain for each additional year of life.   This powder may be repeated, if necessary, every other day for a number of times; and I prefer to have it given in the morning rather than at night, that the effects may be better watched, and that any uneasiness occasioned thereby may not disturb the night's rest. Often the powders need to be given but once or twice a week, and later on only as occasion demands. Any irregularity of the bowels, and especially any tendency to pulmonary congestion, should at once be treated by one of these powders. There is no objection to giving an equivalent quantity of mercury with chalk, but in the main I prefer the action of calomel.

For children a little older in years, a very valuable remedy is a mixture containing rhubarb with soda (Formula 7), given three times daily after meals, in quantities sufficient to act a little upon the bowels. I do not use the more elegant preparations, such as spiced syrup of rhubarb, etc., as I believe them often inferior in efficacy to others which may be less palatable. In the constipation of infants and children connected with eczema, I have had very good results from the frequent and free use of lactopeptine, in doses sufficient to produce the desired effect. This is to be given directly after eating, and may be repeated once or more after each meal if necessary, even in doses of several grains. It is very conveniently administered in suspension, as in orange flower water, though children very often like it dry on the tongue.

Where there is habitual constipation which is not overcome after the bowels have been moderately assisted, other elements must be carefully looked into, such as are indicated elsewhere. The diet must often be changed, and cracked wheat and occasionally oat meal may be added to the food, even of very small infants ; this is best given in the form of a pulp made by rubbing the thoroughly boiled substances through a fine sieve ; also the darker kinds of bread made from whole wheat flour, as mentioned in the chapter on the diet and hygiene.

As in adults, so in infants and children, alkalies are often required, and are of great service in eczema. In nursing infants, I generally give the mother acetate of potassium, ten to fifteen grains three times daily, after eating, with nux vomica and a bitter infusion (Formula 2). I do not know if the potassa passes through the milk, but it certainly benefits the child very much. Where there is a tendency to looseness with windy passages, an alkali may be advantageously administered to the child, combined with chalk mixture and a carminative (Formula 6). Lime water is also of good service given freely to the child, though I do not use it as frequently as many. A good method of administering an alkali, is to dilute the milk with Vichy water, using it rather freely; when the bowels are constipated, Kissingen water may be added in quantities sufficient to relax the bowels a little. Children also do well with a few drops of liquor potassæ added to the milk, from two to five drops in the tumblerful, according to the age. Soda has been suggested as more appropriately agreeing with the normal ingredients of the milk, but I much prefer the action of salts of potassa, both on the stomach and in their effect on the eczema. Magnesia may be used in the same manner, and has the additional advantage of its laxative action.

When there is a good deal of restlessness at night, and the skin is rather dry and hard, the acetate of potassium is of value, given to the child three or four times daily, in doses from one to five grains, in a teaspoonful of the liquor ammoniæ acetatis (Formula 3), with a drop or so of nitre. If there is much arterial excitement, this is improved by the addition of a drop or part of a drop of the tincture of aconite. The extract or tincture of viola tricolor has been recently revived as a remedy in infantile eczema; I have no great experience to offer on the subject, as I have generally found the other measures here recommended to be quite sufficient. The older French writers speak well of it; as it is generally given in connection with senna, so that quite free evacuation of the bowels is induced, it is doubtful how much of the beneficial effect is to be ascribed to the viola, and how much to the senna.

Besides alkalies, cod liver oil, arsenic, and iron, should never be forgotten in infantile eczema. Wine of iron, the ammoniated citrate of iron, tartrate of iron, and dialyzed iron are especially applicable. My most common combination for children contains also a little arsenic (Formula 10); I also make considerable use of the syrup of the hypophosphites of soda, lime, and iron, and am more and more pleased with its effects; also the syrup of the lacto-phosphate of lime. I do not use the syrup of the iodide of iron as much as do some, as I have seen it very often ineffectually employed by others.

Children bear arsenic remarkably well. Some time ago I reported a number of cases of infantile eczema, where the disease yielded in a very short time to Fowler's solution given alone, and since then I have had further proof of its power over the disease. The arsenical solution was given in cinnamon water, and of such a strength that each five or ten drops represented one of the Fowler's solution. This was administered in such a quantity that the child a year old began with a drop of Fowler three times daily, the dose being gradually increased by one-fifth of a drop, until two, three, or even up to ten drops of the arsenical solution were taken with the meals thrice daily, or until there was some diarrhœa; the dose was then lessened. Under this plan the eruption quickly paled in these cases, and soon ceased, with little or no local treatment, and with few if any dietetic or hygienic directions. But I have never felt it wise to recommend this plan, or to practice it very largely, for fear of possible evil results from the free use of so powerful a remedy. I have also seen a number of infants where it had been used previously without effect. While arsenic is given, the necessity of free and natural action of the bowels must be ever kept prominent.

In combination with other measures, arsenic should seldom if ever be neglected in the treatment of eczema in early life, especially in combination with the wine of iron (Formula 10), which mixture much resembles the ferro-arsenical mixture of Mr. Wilson, which he lauds so highly.

It is not a little difficult to express in words, the exact directions for the employment of the various remedies mentioned, and perhaps intelligent judgment will best decide, if it is borne in mind that it is the patient rather than the disease which we have to treat internally. The indications to be followed are those suggested by educated thought directed to restoring the system to perfect health, rather than to special remedies called for by the disease in question.

There are, however. tolerably clear lines of distinction between the class of cases which call for alkaline and depurative treatment, and those where cod liver oil and more powerful tonics are at once demanded. Thus, in the full, ruddy-faced child, with an eczema tending to give a dry, red surface, or perhaps exuding considerable serum when washed or scratched, a full tonic course of treatment will certainly aggravate the complaint, especially if the child comes of gouty stock. In such a case depurative remedies and alkalies will be followed by an amelioration of the itching, a lessening of the cutaneous congestion, and subsidence of the disease. On the other hand, the pale strumous child, in whom the discharge tends to crust up into yellow masses, will be benefited at once by iron, arsenic, cod liver oil, syrup of the hypophosphites, etc. But this latter child, if care be not taken, may soon have the organs of life choked by a sudden influx of material to which it is unaccustomed, and will require the cooling treatment of an occasional purgative, probably also some alkalies. Calomel is better for the first class of patients, and rhubarb and castor oil are better suited for occasional use in the second.

But no hard and fast lines can be laid down ; and there are many cases which cannot be put clearly in either category, but which partake both of the gouty and strumous type. Not infrequently we give tonics and builders up of tissue with one hand while with the other calomel, grey powder, alkalies, etc., are administered. It must also never be forgotten that the full-blooded, arthritic case first described, will at a later period require the tonic course ; for eczema is a disease of debility, whether there is a temporary and false appearance of hyper-activity of the system or not.

While the general measures advised for infantile eczema have not differed so very greatly from those which are required in other conditions, and while emphasis has been laid on the fact that it is the patient rather than the disease which is to be studied for treatment, the local management of the eruption often presents difficulties which demand a special knowledge, experience and care in order to obtain the best results. It is in the local treatment of diseases of the skin, especially in that of eczema, both in infants and in adult life, that wisdom is required to make just the right application ; for the wrong one pretty certainly will not do good, but will positively do harm.

To readily appreciate the necessity for care in regard to local treatment, the physiological conditions of the child's skin, which were previously alluded to, must constantly be borne in mind ; its exceeding delicacy of structure, and the very great proneness to inflammation which it shares in common with all the tissues of infant life, all call for caution in regard to the treatment of it when diseased. The error most commonly made in this, as in all other forms of eczema, is in the direction of too harsh treatment ; the irritable, unprotected skin is too often subjected even to great rudeness. The epithelial layer, whose function it is to receive the wear and tear of the external world, is diseased and often removed, and the inflamed parts below seek to protect themselves by the formation of scales and crusts, which but imperfectly represent the covering belonging to the perfect economy. The part of the medical man is to soothe and protect this inflamed surface, while at the same time the parts are gently urged to healthy action.

The experience both of the special and general medical profession has undoubtedly given to oxide of zinc ointment the palm for universality of use, and that perhaps rightly. But he is poorly able to treat infantile eczema who knows only oxide of zinc ointment; and that as it is directed to be made in the pharmacopœia. The officinal ointment is prepared with lard, with a drachm of tincture of benzoin to the ounce, and eighty grains of oxide of zinc. This I have repeatedly seen irritate tender skins to which, if otherwise prepared, a zinc ointment was soothing. I never use lard in ointments if it can possibly be avoided, my preference being for the cold cream or unguentum aquæ rosæ. This is made from almond oil, spermaceti and beeswax; frequently the odor of the rose is objected to by patients, and the rose-water can be omitted, as it is not an essential ingredient. This cold cream may sometimes become rancid, although it has but a slight tendency thereto : it, as well as other excipients, should be watched, as a rancid oily matter is exceedingly irritating to a diseased skin. The unguentum petrolei, cosmoline or vaseline, or the glycerite of starch is preferable to lard, but the cold cream is really the best of all. The products of petroleum mentioned have not sufficient consistency, when applied they too readily melt and run off, leaving the skin exposed. If any specimen of the cold cream is found too soft, its consistency can be increased by a larger proportion of spermaceti.

The strength of eighty grains of oxide of zinc to the ounce is frequently too great in infantile eczema, and I seldom employ more than sixty grains, and far more often order but thirty grains in each ounce of ointment. I do not benzoate the ointment, as I find this sometimes irritates. In exceedingly sensitive skins I have sometimes found the cucumber ointment, of older writers, more soothing even than the rose ointment.

Bismuth sub-nitrate forms a very good ointment for infantile eczema, used in the strength of half a drachm or a drachm to the ounce. Tannin also acts very happily when there is a dry, red, and somewhat scaly surface. Likewise the ammoniated mercury ointment diluted three or four times with rose-ointment. To relieve the intense itching accompanying the disease, we may, even in the more acute forms of infantile eczema, frequently obtain most excellent results from the addition of a little tar to the ointment, care being taken that the proportion is not too great. The most serviceable mode in which to employ it is by a proper dilution of the old-fashioned tar ointment, a remedy which has fallen into unmerited neglect. Tar ointment as directed by the Pharmacopœia, made of equal parts of tar and suet, is much too strong for application to a child's skin, or to an inflamed surface ; but when diluted with from three to six times its quantity of rose-ointment, with a half drachm or a drachm of oxide zinc in the ounce (Formula 57), it forms one of the most valuable anti-pruritic remedies possible in eczema. Made thus, it can be applied even upon a very young child with the best effects.

In the management of infantile eczema, as in all forms of the complaint, very different results are obtained according to the mode in which the applications are made to the diseased surfaces. In general, ointments should be spread upon cloths and laid upon the affected parts if there is any tendency to exudation. More harm is often done by the efforts of the attendant to rub on the ointment than gain is had from the application itself. If laid on with a cloth, all this is avoided. The dressing should be renewed occasionally, that is with sufficient frequency to secure complete protection of the parts from the air. The first application of any ointment may be resisted by the child, and may seem not to give relief; but if a suitable application has been selected, and if it is renewed as often as it falls off or is brushed off, relief will soon be obtained, and the child who first resisted the application will shortly crave it. This matter of the constant protection, day and night, of eczematous surfaces from the irritating action of the air and external contact, must be insisted upon, and carried out at all hazards, with rigid severity. Attendants will often neglect it, and the application will often be intentionally removed in anticipation of the physician's visit, or when inconvenient on account of ordinary matters of daily life. A single neglect, for even a short period, followed by scratching and irritation of the skin can result in more damage than can be repaired by long treatment.

Powders are not very suitable to infants and children with eczema, even in the more acute stages. They do not afford sufficient relief and protection, and the great tendency to exudation in infantile eczema, renders them powerless to keep the surface dry; consequently a paste will often be formed of the irritating secretion and the powder, especially between folds of skin, as about the neck and groins, which will prove most harmful in eczema of portions of the body where two surfaces of the skin touch one another. The best way to treat these parts is to direct that a piece of muslin, double the size of the diseased patch, be spread thickly with the ointment and then doubled and laid between the parts, so that each diseased surface has the ointment directly in contact with it. Sometimes I have thought that there was much more gain when the cloth had been previously scorched; possibly the gain resulted from the products of combustion, such as creosote, developed in the process, possibly from a destruction of germs which otherwise might exist on the cloth, and excite disease. Carbolic acid is of itself of some little value in infantile eczema, and when added to ointments, a few drops to the ounce, will aid at times in controlling the itching; but it is inferior for this purpose to the tar compound previously spoken of.

Lotions are very little used in infantile eczema, but there is no reason why such soothing applications as are mentioned in connection with acute eczema of other parts of the body (Formulæ 31, 32, 33), should not be of service here as well. The liquor picis alkalinus (Formula 40), diluted twenty or more times with water, will sometimes be found to give very great relief to the pruritus of infantile eczema, as well as in adult life. It should be followed by mild ointment.

In the management of infantile eczema, attention should be always paid to the employment of water by the attendants, for most erroneous methods and ways of using it are constantly practiced, and the existing and continuing cause of eczema in the young, as well as in the old, will not infrequently be found in the abuse of water upon a diseased skin; sometimes also, possibly, in the soap employed. The child with eczema should not be freely washed as if in health, but if washed at all the water should be properly medicated; I generally have the child only wiped off so much as cleanliness actually demands. As a rule, the less washing the better. If a bath is given, a mixture of powdered borax, carbonate of soda, carbonate of potash, made in the proportions of one, two, and three parts may be employed, of which from two to four teaspoonfuls are dissolved in each gallon of bath water, with double the amount of dry starch. This is used without soap, and on taking the child from the bath, it is immediately dried without friction, and the proper medicament at once applied. If there is any tendency to the development of acute papular eczema, or general surface eruption, it should be well powdered all over as with lycopodium or starch powder.

The practice of many is to wash the parts directly affected with eczema; and as .I have learned the advice of the physician, it was to keep the parts well washed and clean. Now it is impossible to keep the surface free from the products of the disease, at least in eczema which is at all acute. As often as the surface is washed, the outer epidermal cells are removed before they have acquired any firmness, a new layer of exudate is immediately formed, and the process is repeated day by day without any tendency to cure, indeed the process of repair is hindered thereby. In localized, chronic, and thickened patches, especially in adults, it is often necessary to wash off the outer imperfectly formed epithelial layers, as described elsewhere, but in acute or sub-acute eczema in infants or small children, this plan is wholly inapplicable. My constant direction is that the eczematous part shall not be washed at all until I direct it to be done; and in many cases this is delayed for a considerable period, and very seldom directed. Occasionally the mass of accumulated secretion becomes so great that the ointment does not penetrate it, and a single washing is of the greatest value in allowing the dressing to come down directly upon the affected surface. This washing may be done, either with the alkaline solution just directed for the bath, or it answers very well to use a good tar soap, or Pear's English transparent soap. But great care must be taken that the operation be not prolonged too greatly, and that the parts are not too much irritated by attempting to remove scales or crusts. I always direct that the application of the ointment shall be made in the quickest time possible after the washing, otherwise a coat of exudate has formed and hardened, and the medicament lies on top of it, and fails of its end.

In young children I seldom have parts which are at all acutely involved in the eczematous process washed more than once or twice a week; sometimes not at all for a much longer time. When the crusts are very thick, as upon the scalp, we have a very valuable agent to penetrate them in cod liver oil, whose value as a local application in eczema is by no means small. Its efficacy is often much increased by the addition of a small portion of oil of cade to it, say one part in from eight to sixteen (Formula 49), especially if there is much itching.

A word may here be said in reference to the use of poultices in infantile eczema. In the more than six hundred cases of eczema in children under five years of age, which are here analyzed I believe that I can count on the fingers of my hands, the number of poultices which have been applied under my direction. I almost never order them, and yet it is the commonest thing to hear of others directing them to be used, and, I believe, generally to the detriment of the case. Occasionally when there is a thick crust which refuses to come away with ointment or oil, a single poultice may be applied for the night and the crust removed in the morning, and the appropriate ointment at once reapplied. Sometimes a second poultice may be required, but very rarely more than this; and I never have the scalp or other eczematous surface treated continuously with poultices, as is frequently advised.

When eczema has lost its very acute elements, or when under such treatment as has been mentioned, we find that it refuses to yield, we may, as in the adult, resort to stimulation ; and this if applied correctly will often furnish the best results. The tar-ointment previously alluded to may be increased in strength even up to almost equal quantities of the officinal tar ointment and rose ointment with half a drachm or a drachm of zinc or bismuth in the ounce. Or we may find very much benefit from the use of zinc ointment with a drachm or more of the oil of cade or the oil of birch rubbed in it, (Formula 58). Where there is much itching, the addition to an ointment of a drachm of the tincture of camphor, or a few grains of powdered camphor in the ounce will often give relief, but it must be used with some caution in children. In patches which are more chronic and rebellious we will often get most benefit from one of the mercurial ointments, and I use a good deal of the unguentum hydragyri oxidi rubri, diluted with three times its quantity or more of rose ointment (Formula 66). But this I have repeatedly found to be too strong, exciting a fresh papular eruption for which a milder treatment must be at once employed. The citrine ointment diluted three, four, or more times, is also of service where patches are chronic and non-inflammatory. The compound ointment of acetate of lead and mercury (Formula 68), is used greatly in England in the treatment of eczema of children ; it is a little stimulating, but generally is well borne. These stronger ointments employed in more chronic and rebellious patches, find their value in being rather rubbed into the skin, and not simply applied upon muslin or lint as directed in the more acute stages.

The compound tincture of green soap of Hebra, composed of equal parts of the oil of cade, green soap, and alcohol, is often times of great value if carefully applied in the eczema of young children. It may be employed in full strength, but generally it is better to dilute it a little with water at the time of using, certainly the first time it is applied to any surface ; for with eczema one can never be

sure even that a remedy which has proved serviceable in
other cases will not irritate some particular skin. It is to
be quickly but firmly rubbed on, with a cloth dampened
in it, and the part is then gently dried off or even bathed
off quickly with water, and the proper ointment immediately applied. It is a most valuable antipruritic remedy,
and will at times arrest the itching excellently. When
this is used it is far' better always to have the suitable
ointment, which should be of the mildest kind, spread on
a rag and laid on, as the extra friction of any application
with the fingers or otherwise may be just so much more
than the skin requires.

In this chapter I have by no means exhausted all that
could be said upon the subject of the management of infantile eczema, but I have endeavored to lay down the
principles upon which the treatment of the disease must
be based in order to be successful. In no class of cases
is it so necessary to bear in mind the value of proper
soothing treatment, as in eczema occurring in infants and
small children. And yet, in certain instances where the
eruption is chronic and rebellious, the most varied and
often severe measures can be applied with benefit and.
safety, but this is comparatively rare. In more chronic
cases where the eruption has lasted from the earliest life
for months, or several years, the eruption partakes more
of the character belonging to eczema of older life ; and
further principles for its guidance may be found in other
chapters relating to eczema of special regions.
It has been the aim of this chapter not only to furnish
details in regard to the local management of infantile eczema, but to impress the fact that we have to do, not with
a local disease of the skin alone, but with one intimately
connected with and dependent on other causes than the
outward irritation which apparently may have given rise

to the eruption.　To rightly cure infantile eczema, all the elements of the child's health must be studied and understood, and intelligent therapy will embrace not only the remedies and measures that may be appropriate to the skin manifestations present, but every element capable of having any effect upon the child's health and well-being.

A single further clinical observation may be added in proof of the constitutional nature of the disease, which while not established with absolute certainty, is yet of sufficient interest to demand further investigation and thought. Among very many instances where the matter has been inquired into, I have found that infants with eczema have not been in the habit of bringing up or throwing off the food, but have been 'often noted as being very " dry babies"; whereas on the contrary, I have rarely met with a child who raised the milk much, who was troubled to any degree, if at all, with eczema.　I have also very frequently remarked that in a family of children, all the " wet babies," who have rejected milk from the stomach, have been free from eczema, while others nursing the same mother, but who have retained all their food, have frequently suffered from the disease.　The relief to the system from the acid ejected from the stomach, has seemed to spare them from the acid blood state which is believed to exist with eczema.　Possibly the immunity of " wet babies" may be explained by the relief to the organs of digestion afforded by the rapid rejection of food which would otherwise be in excess, and thus lead to imperfect carrying out of the processes of assimilation and disintegration of tissue.

CHAPTER X.

SOME of the most troublesome and rebellious cases of eczema are those in which the face and scalp are affected, and not infrequently the eruption will yield on every other portion of the body and linger here long afterwards, seeming almost to defy complete cure; while not at all infrequently these parts are affected alone from first to last.

The reasons for the obstinacy of eczema in the regions under consideration are several, which it is well always to bear in mind in the management of these cases. First, the eruption is almost invariably directly connected with dyspeptic conditions, often those which are very manifest and rebellious, but perhaps almost as often with those which are hidden and difficult to reach. In addition to the general systemic causes resulting from this indigestion, as detailed in other chapters, there is a reflex nervous influence exerted directly from the digestive organs upon these parts, which seems to act very promptly and powerfully in augmenting eczema in this location. Eczema of these regions, as likewise that upon the hands, is also often seen to be remarkably affected by general nervous conditions, each excitement, depression or exhaustion being followed by fresh outbreaks or by an aggravation of an existing eruption, as in the instances cited in the chapter on the causes of eczema.

Another reason for the obstinacy of the eruption of eczema in this locality, especially upon the face, lies undoubtedly in the local irritants to which the surfaces are continually exposed.   The first of these to be considered is the irritation of motion from the impossibility of keeping the parts at rest.   Chronic eczema about the mouth is peculiarly rebellious to treatment, owing to the incessant movements occurring here, and the same applies to almost every portion of the region under consideration.   Another disadvantageous element, is the readiness with which the eruption is reached for scratching, and the almost irresistible tendency which exists to touch it, with the occurrence of any uncomfortable feeling.   Furthermore there is considerable difficulty in making exactly proper applications to this portion of the body and of keeping them continuously in position; this trouble often arises from the patient being unwilling to keep the dressings upon the parts all the time until the disease is absolutely and entirely removed.   Thus the eruption gets almost well, and the treatment is neglected to a greater or less degree. and as a consequence local influences again excite the disease to fresh development.

The local irritating agencies which operate especially on the face and scalp, are many and varied.   First, we have the continual exposure to air which results from the repeated and frequent removal of the applications, which pertains to these more than to any other parts of the body; this often occurs accidentally, as in wiping the face, friction with the bed-clothes, etc., but is also voluntary in many instances, as, when the patient without permission will be content with covering and protecting the surface only at night, or removes the applications temporarily when going into the society of others.

In addition to the harm from the contact of the air, we have also the irritation resulting from changes of temperature and humidity, which, it can be easily understood, affect these exposed regions of the body much more readily and actively than those which are naturally protected. It is not at all uncommon to see eczema of the face and ears made very much worse after exposure to the sun, as when out boating or driving, or after a walk in a cutting or chilling wind; also after exposure to artificial heat, as over the fire, in cooking, etc.

Next, water is far more apt to be applied to these parts, even when diseased, than to other portions of the body, and this is an element of irritation which the physician will find it most difficult to reach; the idea of not washing the face repeatedly is so repugnant to many, that it is next to impossible to prevent much harm being done thus to the eruption, either without or with a guarded permission.

Too frequent, severe, or prolonged cleansing of the scalp, either with the comb or brush, or by washing, will excite and also render very obstinate an eruption of eczema located there, and I have seen many instances where the main obstacle to cure was too great washing, even such as was directed by the physician.

The constant exposure of the face, scalp and ears, also results in the lodgment upon the skin of much dust, and often of particles which are particularly obnoxious; smoking is frequently the cause of great aggravation of eczema of the face by the direct irritation of the smoke, as well as by its general and nervous effect upon the disease, as more particularly mentioned elsewhere.

Certain cases of eczema of the face, as well as of the hands, have their origin in poisoning by the rhus toxicodendron or poison ivy or oak, and the impression left on tissues may continue for a great length of time; and further, there may occur fresh irritation with each returning season, and the eruption may be thus prolonged for years. I have known cases where even riding through a region thickly infested with the plant, during certain seasons, would cause great aggravation of an eczema which had laid dormant, perhaps, for months.

Other possible local irritants must be ever borne in mind in the management of these cases, or they may prove wholly rebellious to even the best measures. I have seen a hat band, probably containing a poisonous dye, cause the eruption on the forehead on several occasions. Irritating soap has repeatedly given rise to eczema of the hands and face, and in one instance where the eruption recurred repeatedly after shaving with a certain soap, the latter was found on microscopic examination to contain minute spiculæ of bone, and when its use was discontinued the eruption ceased. Too close shaving, a dull razor, bad after-treatment of the skin, etc., can all excite and prolong an eruption of eczema on the face.

It will be thus seen that there are abundant and good reasons for the obstinacy of the eruption in the locations under consideration, and a successful management of the disease involves attention to these and to others which may have escaped mention.

The diagnosis of eczema of the face and scalp need not generally give much trouble, but in some cases it presents very great difficulty. The appearances which the eruption assumes on these parts are most varied, and to those unaccustomed to the disease individual cases may appear so vastly different from each other that it would hardly be supposed that they were instances of the same affection. It will be necessary therefore to bear well in mind what was said in the chapters upon the lesions and the forms of eczema, and upon diagnosis.

All the lesions and forms of eczema may be seen on the face and scalp, although the erythematous and pustular conditions are more common in adults. The phases of the eruption in these locations in infants and children have been described in the chapter on infantile eczema, and need not be detailed here.

Eczema may manifest itself upon the hairy scalp in

three quite distinct forms of eruption ; the pustular, the moist exuding, and the dry scaly. Pustular or impetiginous eczema of the scalp is more often seen in young persons than in those of older life ; in infants it forms what is known as milk crust, as described in the previous chapter, which condition may occasionally last from infancy even to youth or longer. Generally some perfect pustules can be seen in the scalp in those of older years, although often only small crusts are found, adherent to the hairs, and beneath them raw and moist points ; these are observed to be very superficial, and on healing do not leave scars. As a rule eczema exists elsewhere at the same time, especially behind and above the ears, or on the face. In severe cases the pustules run more or less together and the pus dries into masses which become matted together among the hairs, into greenish-yellow crusts; these may become blackened by dust or blood, and the scalp then presents a loathsome appearance with a sickening odor. The inflammation prevents a proper care of the hair, it cannot be combed or dressed, and sometimes these cases are so long neglected that the entangled hair, crusts, and sebaceous secretion form a dense mass, which then attracts lice, which in turn add to the repulsive condition. This uncared for condition of the scalp still further invites the presence of vegetable parasites and the combined state almost defies description. It was to this condition that the name of *Plica Polonica* was formerly given, and in Vienna I have seen these neglected cases where the mass of hair, etc., had become so matted and hardened that it sounded like a board when rapped on. Happily such cases are unknown among the more enlightened classes. Pustular eczema does not usually itch much, but the advent of pediculi will cause this to occur.

Pustular eczema of the scalp must be differentiated from simple phthiriasis capitis which need not be a true eczema; that is, this latter is simply an inflammatory action in the skin, or a dermatitis, wholly due to the irritation of lice and the consequent scratching, though the lesions often resemble those of eczema very closely. Often a very few lice will occasion and keep up the eruption, and unless this cause is recognized and removed the case will resist all ordinary treatment.

In cleanly persons who have pediculi the scalp may be examined again and again without discovering any of the insects, for they are frequently removed by washing or combing. But a careful search will always detect their eggs or nits adhering to the hairs, sometimes several in a row on a hair, more commonly only one; the most usual seat of the nit is about one inch from the scalp. The scales in squamous eczema will occasionally resemble these nits very closely, when they are scattered as dandruff through the hair, but the difference may be readily established by the loose, movable character of the scale and the hard, immovable position of the nit.

The eruption from lice is far more common among females than among males, and generally the preponderance of the lesions is found on the back and lower part of the scalp, where the insects find warmth and protection beneath the larger mass of hair there collected. There are no absolute differences which can be described between the lesions occurring in ordinary pustular eczema of the scalp and those caused by lice. But there are general distinctions which should be borne in mind. The pustules of true eczema are more decided, and are apt to surround hair follicles, and there is considerable tenderness of the scalp; whereas, in pediculosis the itching is the prominent symptom, and the lesions are the direct result of the scratching or tearing off the crusts time and again. The eruption of pustular eczema of the scalp is more inclined to be general, than in that from lice.

In connection with both pustular eczema and phthiriasis capitis we may have enlarged glands at the back of the neck and behind the ears. These appear to be due to lymphatic absorption from the diseased surfaces, and they vary in size with the severity of the affection and the health of the individual. They seldom give much if any pain, and are of little importance, although parents are often very anxious about them ; they very rarely inflame or suppurate. I do not think I have ever seen one suppurate among scores of cases in which I have observed them. They are quite distinct from the cutaneous abscesses described in connection with infantile eczema.

Pustular syphilis of the scalp sometimes resembles a pustular eczema very closely, and great care may be required to establish the correct diagnosis ; usually other signs of syphilis appear in connection with the early papulo-pustular eruption upon the scalp, which is commonly but a part of a general eruption. In the later pustulo-tubercular eruption, which sometimes attacks the scalp alone, the crusts may resemble those of eczema exactly : but in this syphilitic eruption there is ulceration beneath, and it is followed by cicatrization, which is not the case in eczema, however severe. The odor from the syphilitic eruption is much more apt to be fetid, while that of eczema is nauseous.

The crusts of favus may resemble those of pustular eczema, especially when the favus masses have become heaped together and mingled with inflammatory products resulting from scratching. But somewhere there can usually be found one or more of the typical, cup-shaped masses of favus, which will present the sulphur-yellow color ; and the mass of crusts will always be of a more yellow color than those of eczema, which have a greenish tint. They will also be found to be very friable, crumbling to dust very easily as compared with the crusts from eczema, which, being of inflammatory origin, although they may be crushed readily, will still remain in small masses, not easily yielding. The hairs are peculiarly dry and lustre- less in favus, and generally patches of cicatricial tissue can be seen in cases of much duration, or bare spots, reddened and shiny. When the crusts of favus are gently raised they will be found to be lifted easily from a slightly depressed base which is of a bright red color, shiny, and apparently moist; but no exudation occurs, and what is seen is only the bared rete malpighii and papillary layer, and not an inflammatory surface exuding serum or pus. Finally the microscope shows the crusts of favus to be composed almost entirely of the spores and mycelium of the parasite, while those from eczema show a confused mass of epithelial and exudation elements.

The next variety of eczema of the scalp is the moist or exuding form. In this we do not often find separate vesicles, but when first seen there will be larger or smaller surfaces on which there is a moist secretion, which is found to stiffen the hairs as though mucilage had been applied, and if left alone it will dry into scales or crusts, which latter are less thick and yellow than those pre- viously described in the pustular variety. But there are no well marked lines of distinction between the two, for an eczema may present pustules in one place and serous ex- udation in another, and be dry and scaly in a third, and may also exhibit one or the other at different times. More commonly large surfaces of the scalp are involved in moist eczema, and not at all infrequently the entire region will be the seat of an eruption, which will also extend to the parts behind the ears, or on to the forehead; or not in- frequently an eruption exists elsewhere on the body. This moist form of the eruption is very apt to pass soon into the next variety, namely the scaly, and they will therefore be spoken of together.

Squamous or scaly eczema, or, named after the lesion,

erythematous eczema, exhibits many different phases and degrees, from an insignificant dry scaling, giving annoyance principally by the dust shed on the clothing, to an intensely itchy and distressing condition, exhibiting at one time moisture, at another thick, scaly crusts, which are very manifest. This scaly state may exist either independently of other apparent disease, that is, not having been preceded by moisture, or it may be the later stage of an exuding vesicular or pustular eczema.

In the milder states, coming on gradually, without any inflammatory period, it forms a large share of the cases exhibiting what is popularly called dandruff or dandriff; this often lasts for years, giving comparatively little annoyance, until perhaps some violent cleansing of the scalp, or some irritating hair wash excites a condition of inflammation, and a readily recognized eczema is developed. It may perchance happen that the same irritation has sufficed only to keep up a moderate degree of scaling, until internal causes, debility, etc. have rendered them operative to a greater degree, and inflammation results.

This form of eczema of the scalp is accompanied with considerable itching, but seldom to the degree exhibited by the eruption in other localities; there is not infrequently considerable soreness, and tenderness on pressure.

There is a form of erythematous eczema appearing at the nape of the neck, extending both among the hairs, sometimes to considerable distance, and down the neck even on to the shoulders, which deserves special mention because of its obstinacy. It may exist with an eruption of eczema elsewhere, or it may be present as the sole manifestation of the disease. The surface is reddened, and roughened with a moderate amount of scales; papules are seldom seen, and rarely moisture, unless a little appears after scratching. There is decided infiltration or thickening, and the margin of the eruption is generally pretty sharply defined, but the patch is irregular in shape, and not composed of separate spots as in psoriasis. The itching of the eruption in this location is a very marked and often an exceedingly annoying symptom, and the condition sometimes proves very rebellious.

There are a number of eruptions which closely resemble dry eczema upon the scalp; they are seborrhœa, tinea tonsurans, psoriasis, pityriasis capitis, and favus, named in the order of their probable frequency of presentation for diagnosis.

Seborrhœa may be distinguished from eczema, by the more greasy character of the scales, which tend to adhere to the scalp, although they also become loosened and dry, and may fall on the clothing in dandruff like those of eczema. Seborrhœa never gives the history of exudation; it itches very moderately, if at all; the skin beneath is generally rather more pale than normal, instead of being reddened as in eczema; and, in seborrhœa the whole scalp or areas of considerable size are generally affected quite uniformly, whereas differences in degree can commonly be made out in eczema. The eruption of seborrhœa elsewhere, if it is not confined to the hairy scalp, occurs on places where sebaceous glands are abundant, as on the nose, cheeks, and chest, whereas very commonly eczema appears indifferently elsewhere, as well as on the scalp.

Recent cases of tinea tonsurans, with their circular patches, on which there is broken hair, can hardly be mistaken for eczema. But when the eruption of ringworm has lasted for some time, and a large surface is involved, and when the hairs have grown tolerably well in spite of the disease, the real nature of the eruption may be easily overlooked, and it may pass for scaly eczema. Here, however, a little careful examination will readily cause suspicion, and the microscope will demonstrate the fungus, if the eruption be parasitic. In this case the surface is of a dull leaden color, with a considerable amount of dirty scaling, and close examination will reveal broken hairs amid the longer ones; in ringworm the hairs either come out easily when extracted, or break off, and the fringed or brush-like end of the hair, with the spores and mycelium of the parasite, may be readily made out by the microscope. The stubbed hairs can generally be felt, by passing the fingers lightly over the surface at a little distance from the skin.

Psoriasis frequently exists on the scalp alone, and may cause much desquamation, the scales falling as dandruff. But psoriasis on the scalp exhibits the same features as elsewhere, namely separate patches or spots of various sizes, generally round, with scales on a reddened base. Eczema is seen in larger patches, irregular, and with illy-defined margins, shading off gradually into the healthy skin. Psoriasis is always a dry disease from first to last, and even when the scales are scraped off and slight bleeding results, the surface will not exude, but dries over with a new formation of scale, or at most with a slightly bloody crust. The scales of psoriasis are far more apt to adhere in masses, and to come off in heaped up plates, covering even a patch of some size; those of eczema if not exudative, are either dry and branny, or adherent in single, larger scales, and not micaceous and in layers as in psoriasis. The itching of psoriasis is always much less than that of eczema, and there is no general thickening or infiltration of the skin such as is seen in the latter. Very commonly sooner or later psoriasis will show itself characteristically elsewhere.

Pityriasis capitis resembles the scaly stage of eczema, but differs from it essentially in its course and symptoms; although some writers have failed to distinguish between the two affections. In pityriasis we have simply an excessive exfoliation and shedding of the epidermal cells, with perhaps slight reddening of the skin, and very moderate itching, if any.   In more severe cases the epithelial masses are seen to extend around and embrace quite firmly the hairs in the form of a small sheath, and many of these may be seen on the hairs at different points, detached from the surface of the scalp.   The process here, as in psoriasis, is always a dry one, and the whole or a greater part of the scalp, and often the beard also, is involved.

Favus has been mentioned as being possibly liable to be mistaken for the pustular form of eczema of the scalp. In old cases we sometimes have a mild, scaly condition in favus, which may resemble eczema squamosum of the scalp.   But the dry, lustreless condition and thinness of the hair, and the history of the case should excite suspicion, and generally one or more crusts, more or less characteristic of favus, can be found ; in cases which have arrived at this stage, there has generally more or less cicatrization already taken place.   Moreover, microscopic examination of the scales, crusts, and hairs, shows the presence of the vegetable parasite.

Eczema of the face may assume any or all of the features of the disease, and the forms and appearances in different cases may be so greatly varied as hardly to be recognized to be the same eruption by those unfamiliar with the disease.

The face is a very common seat of the eruption in infants, as mentioned in the preceding chapter.   In young persons it is not at all uncommon to have eczema take a pustular form about the mouth, nose or chin, with or without an eruption elsewhere ; this, which is often called impetiginous eczema, corresponds to the impetigo of older writers.   Here it appears as patches of inflamed skin covered with greenish-yellow scabs, which latter reform as often as removed, and beneath these there is found a moist, exuding surface.

Acute eczema in older persons generally takes the papular and vesicular form, although in some localities the erythematous variety will also appear very acutely, as for instance, about the eyes; this will be described more minutely with chronic erythematous eczema, which is its most usual form.

Acute papulo-vesicular eczema of the face should not present much difficulty of diagnosis. We observe in it groups of papules or vesicles, closely set, often in more or less circular patches, with a very considerable amount of burning and stinging pain, and seldom with any itching at the outset. The papules and vesicles soon become covered with small scaly crusts, which, when removed, are found to cover shotty papules which may then remain for some time and be very itchy. Sometimes the eczematous patches are more or less circular, presenting an evenly reddened, papular surface, and might then possibly be confounded with ringworm of the face; in the latter, however, we have one or more circular spots, which begin from small points and enlarge peripherally, while they tend to clear in the centre, whereas the eczematous patches are generally more marked in the centre and less developed on the circumference, and do not give the history of a gradual peripheral increase. Sometimes the diagnosis is very difficult, but a few days will generally suffice to clear up the matter, the course of the two eruptions being very different; the trichophyton can usually be demonstrated in the ringworm without much difficulty.

Acute pustular eczema is not very uncommon upon parts of the face covered with hair; and here it sometimes persists with amazing obstinacy. There are only four or five conditions which could be mistaken for eczema in this region; these are, ringworm, tinea barbæ, or parasitic sycosis; true, non-parasitic sycosis; acne; syphilis; and epithelioma. If the essential features and real character of eczema be borne in mind the diagnosis is usually easy. In regard to the differentiation of pustular eczema of the face from ringworm, parasitic sycosis, or barber's itch, it is to be remembered that eczema is an inflammatory affection, and that the pustules are the result of the intensity of the inflammation; in it we generally have considerable superficial redness and swelling and infiltration of the part, with a greater or less production of pustules and consequent crusting. In ringworm of the bearded face the history of a development from a small point or several points, with a gradual peripheral spreading in more or less circular form can be made out, and not at all infrequently the distinct line or margin of the ring can be seen, even when there is an inflammatory and pustular eruption from the parasite. In the parasitic disease crusts are not abundant, if indeed there are any, while in eczema the tendency is toward pus formation and the consequent matting of crusts among the hairs. If there are inflamed masses in tinea sycosis they are boggy elevations of some size, uneven on their surface, and the hairs will be found to stand loose in their follicles, and are generally extracted without pain. In eczema the hairs are firmly seated, even when pus has formed around them, and there is exquisite pain when traction is made upon them; when they are drawn out the roots are found covered with inflammatory products in a large succulent mass, presenting a different appearance from the dark, dull, unhealthy character of those in tinea sycosis, which usually come out without their root sheaths, if the disease has advanced to suppuration.

The differentiation between true or non-parasitic sycosis, and pustular eczema of the hairy parts is occasionally very difficult; indeed, sycosis sometimes appears to be of eczematous origin. But there are differential points which are generally sufficiently marked to admit of an exact diagnosis. Sycosis being a disease of the hair follicles, or rather a peri-folliculitis, the eruption is necessarily confined to the hairy parts, whereas in eczema the eruption will very frequently be found to extend on to parts not covered with hair. When pustules are formed in sycosis the pus has already burrowed from the bottom, and consequently has detached the hair, so that it stands in the centre of a little well of pus, and may be extracted almost if not quite without pain : when a pustule forms in eczema of the hairy part it is much more superficial, and the hair which may stand in its centre, as in sycosis, is found to be attached firmly at its deeper portion, and traction on it causes great pain. In eczema we are apt to have much more crusting and matting together of the hair than in true sycosis, in which latter the pustules are far more apt to stand isolated, the hairs becoming affected separately and often those at some distance from each other; while in eczema a crop of papules or pustules generally develop all at once, in one locality. Eczema being an affair primarily of the more superficial portion of the skin. it does not destroy the life of the hair, and therefore is not followed by cicatrices ; whereas, sycosis, beginning in the deepest structures, disorganizes first the papilla of the hair, and converts its follicle into a pustule along its entire depth ; the process is then necessarily followed by a new deposit of cicatricial tissue, and this feature in some cases becomes terribly marked and disfiguring. Eczema of the hairy parts itches, often very annoyingly ; with sycosis there is rather a deep feeling of burning pain, increased by handling the hairs.

Acne of bearded parts sometimes resembles pustular eczema, but its presence elsewhere, the isolated and discrete character of the pustules, the presence of soreness in them, and the absence of itching. are sufficient to distinguish it.

A pustular or tubercular eruption of syphilis in the

hairy portions of the face may sometimes be mistaken for eczema; but a consideration of the features of the two, together with what has been said in this connection in reference to the hairy scalp, will prevent mistakes.

Certain cases of superficial epithelioma about the face, are occasionally mistaken for eczema, as I have seen on a number of occasions; but the course and characters of the two should be sufficient to differentiate them. Beneath the little crust which forms in epithelioma, a slightly raw surface is found, which always bleeds very readily, generally even on the removal of the covering.

The most common form in which eczema affects the face, is one in which it is least frequently recognized and appreciated, namely as eczema erythematosum. In this erythematous eczema there are generally no papules, no vesicles, no pustules, but simply an evenly reddened surface, smooth or slightly scaly, with a certain degree of thickening or infiltration, and with intolerable itching; and sometimes with burning and pricking. This condition may affect all or the greater part of the face, or may be confined to definite and circumscribed areas. The most common seats of it are the forehead and eyebrows, lips and chin, and also the nose, either over its whole surface, or only at the angles of its junction with the cheeks. It may occur as an acute, sub-acute or chronic condition; occasionally with a long standing erythematous eczema, there may be a sudden lighting up of the eruption very acutely in some particular place, as about the eyelids, by means of which the eyes may even be closed. Sometimes this erythematous eczema is attended with slight moisture on its surface, this is especially observable on the eyelids; but generally the affected skin is dry and harsh and leathery, presenting to the touch a very striking contrast to the neighboring portion of healthy skin, with its supple, slightly oily feeling.

This form of eczema is most commonly confounded with erysipelas, indeed very many of the cases which I have seen have previously been so regarded. But if the essential features of erysipelas are borne in mind, the mistake need not be made. Erysipelas is an acute disease, and cannot present such a picture as has been described; there is no such a disease as a chronic erysipelas, except in the migratory form which may traverse large areas again and again, but does not remain in a chronic state in one locality. In erysipelas we have the fever, headache, and general constitutional symptoms; the skin is hot, tense, and shiny, and of a much more vivid red than in eczema.

Acne rosacea may sometimes be mistaken for slightly papular and erythematous eczema, especially when this affects the nose, chin, and middle part of the face. But acne being a sebaceous disease, we have in it a greasy condition of skin in place of the dry, harsh state pertaining to this form of eczema, where the sebaceous secretion seems to be almost if not quite arrested. Moreover there will probably be some comedones, painful pustules, or enlarged veins, or other marks pointing to acne, and there will be an absence of the infiltration and itching which always characterize eczema of the face. But in rare cases the two may be confounded, unless considerable care be exercised, and it is also possible for both eruptions to exist together.

The slightly developed erythematous eczema, which sometimes attacks the region at the junction of the nose and cheeks, occasionally passes long unrecognized. Here we have a chronic red surface, quite itchy, and that is about all; there is some thickening, but this is difficult to determine in this location, and there may be a little scaling, but this is kept down by washing; and on account of the very great numbers and size of the sebaceous glands in this locality, the skin is not as dry and harsh as in ery-thematous eczema of other parts. The itching, and red-ness, together with the exclusion of other affections, afford the basis for a differential diagnosis.

The lips are sometimes the seat of very obstinate ec-zema. Pustular eczema of the space beneath the nostrils is not uncommon, both in the hairy lip and on those not covered with hair; here it often depends upon an irri-tating secretion from the nose, and special treatment to the nasal cavity must be given in order to affect a perma-nent cure. This eczema upon the middle portion of the hairy lip sometimes proves most annoying and obstinate; it will almost yield to treatment, and then break out again and again with every accession of a fresh catarrhal cold, or it may disappear entirely with each summer and recur with the advent of cold weather.

The vermilion portion of the lips may also, in rare instances, be affected with eczema to a very annoying degree. Here the surface is of a more brilliant red than normal, is more or less fissured, has ragged epider-mal scales, and is the seat of considerable burning and itching; when wiped dry it may often be observed to ex-ude from many points. This condition may extend to the mucous membrane of the mouth, though this is very rare, and occasion much suffering. From the manner in which this tissue may be affected in this location, the question arises how far the mucous membrane in general may become the seat of eczema, or indeed, of states simi-lar to other affections of the skin; some writers have already spoken of psoriasis of the intestine, and there is reason for believing that certain attacks of asthmatic breathing are due to a condition of the bronchial mucous membrane similar to urticaria. On the interior of the mouth it is difficult to distinguish eczema from certain other lesions which are liable to occur there, especially from those of syphilis. But eczema generally involves a large surface if at all; there is not the pearly appearance seen in syphilis, there is more rawness and a general ragged character of the epidermis, and close observation will sometimes detect points which may well be supposed to be the remains of vesicles. There are few if any diseases which can be confounded with eczema of the lips; febrile herpes is characterized by little groups of vesicles, with a burning, hot, tender feeling; mucous patches are as a rule much more clearly defined and sharply outlined than eczema, and if their well known characters are closely studied, there need be little danger of mistaking the two.

Eczema of the nares, and of the lining membrane of the nose, is sometimes a troublesome affection. One or both nostrils will be thickened and reddened, and patchy crusts will form within the orifice, which reform as often as removed by picking; and if neglected, especially in children, this condition may increase until the nose is completely blocked up, and it and the lips become the seat of a crusted eczema which is repulsive and distressing. In slighter cases the mucous membrane of the nose presents a reddened and raw appearance, with more or less moisture, or it may be glazed over with a dry coating of exudate, or there may be crusts of some considerable extent within the nose. The only lesions which can at all resemble eczema at the orifice of the nose, are some of those of syphilis; in this, however, papules or tubercles generally form, and occasionally mucous patches; in syphilis there is an absence of the exudation and of the itching, and of all the inflammatory phenomena of eczema.

Eczema of the edges of the eyelids may exist as an independent affair or may occur in connection with the same on other portions of the body. It forms quite a large proportion of the cases ordinarily spoken of as blepharitis, and unless attention is paid to constitutional measures such cases may prove exceedingly obstinate, recurring again and again, as often as removed by local treatment. This condition is much more common in children than in adults and especially in those exhibiting a scrofulous state or habit. The edges of the lids, more especially the upper lids, are reddened, swollen, thickened and somewhat itchy; small crusts are seen between the eyelashes, and a considerable tendency always exists to have the eyelids glued together after sleep by the discharge which takes place. This state of the lids does not usually cause as much annoyance as might be expected, except from its appearance, although patients thus affected generally complain to a greater or lesser extent of having " weak eyes." This condition has frequently been called, or rather known as, tinea tarsi ; the name, however, is entirely inapplicable to this state, inasmuch as the term tinea is now accepted as a general one to indicate the vegetable parasitic affections, and the eruption under consideration has nothing whatever to do with any parasite, animal or vegetable. True tinea tarsi is a rare affection, and is not as a rule conjoined with the amount of inflammation which is seen in eczema of this region ; it is generally associated with parasitic disease elsewhere, and the parasite can be demonstrated in the hairs and scales by the microscope. Occasionally pediculi attack the surface of the lids, and give rise to very considerable irritation and itching, and the scratching resulting therefrom may in turn give rise to lesions resembling eczema. This, however, is also rare and usually a little careful observation will show the nits upon the hairs, or the pediculi themselves if they are present.

Eczema of the face is very frequently preceded by or accompanied with styes or hordeoli ; indeed, so very common is it for the meibomian glands to become inflamed in eczematous subjects in general, that I have come to look upon repeated styes as a greater or less indication of the existence of the eczematous state. They are very often promptly checked by the same line of management as serviceable in eczema and furunculi.

Eczema of the ears and neighboring parts is far more common in children than in adults, but is still seen not infrequently both alone, and in connection with eczema of other regions, in persons of all ages. Very often the eruption may be exceedingly slight, confined entirely to a small fissure above, below, or behind the ear, which will almost heal, but open now and again with a little movement of the ear; and from time to time the eruption may extend from this, until a large surface is involved. The region directly behind the ear or above it is far more commonly affected than the ear itself, and the condition seen here is usually that of a slightly .moist, exuding surface which may become more or less covered with scales or crusts. The eruption here varies very greatly in different cases, from the slight fissure before referred to, up to one involving even a large portion of the scalp or neck. Eczema of the auricle may be either acute or chronic; we may have a sudden lighting up of inflammation, generally papular or vesicular, though sometimes only erythematous, and the ear becomes red, swollen, and the seat of severe burning and stinging sensations. The inflammation may extend even into the external meatus which it may close, and cause temporary deafness. Chronic eczema of the auricle is more commonly seen in the papulovesicular form, conjoined with general redness, considerable infiltration, and more or less itching. But itching is not a characteristic or constant symptom of eczema in the region under consideration.

Chronic eczema of the external auditory meatus is not a very uncommon condition, and its real nature is very frequently overlooked. It often lasts for years, giving rise to more or less itching, some little desquamation, and a greater or less degree of deafness. The canal may from time to time fill up with wax and epithelial debris, which are removed once and again by syringing, but return and cause constant annoyance. In certain of these cases a vegetable parasite can be demonstrated, but it is questionable if it is not generally if not always an accidental matter, the primary disease being a low grade of eczematous inflammation, in which the chance parasite finds a ready soil.

The only diseases which are likely to be confounded with eczema of the ear, are erythema, erysipelas, and lupus erythematosus. Erythema simplex sometimes attacks the ears, quite constantly producing some redness and swelling, together with a tingling; but there is an absence of the papules or vesicles, and the subsequent exudation and infiltration seen in eczema; in some instances it is quite impossible to make the diagnosis at once with positiveness. The same is true with regard to erysipelas which attacks the ears not very infrequently. But the progress of the case will generally decide its true nature within a day or so at the most; also concomitant signs will generally assist in determining quite promptly. Certain cases of lupus erythematosus of and about the ears are very difficult of diagnosis from patches of chronic eczema. But they will be found to be of a very chronic character, remaining exactly the same for months or years, exhibiting dry, hardened patches of greater or less extent, sometimes slightly elevated above the level, with a small amount of scales, very firmly adherent, and generally showing on their surface the opening of sebaceous glands filled with a hardened epithelial debris. There is generally no itching, and no inconvenience from the patches of lupus erythematosus, and patients are sometimes unconscious of their existence unless their attention has been called to them by others or by the appearance of the eruption elsewhere, or by having felt the rough-ened skin.

The management of eczema of the region of the scalp and face involves many points, as stated in the opening of the chapter. The eruption in this location is very fre-quently connected with disturbances of the digestive functions, and also very frequently dependent upon nerv-ous causes. The greatest care will therefore be neces-sary in investigating the internal relations of these cases, and in removing in every possible way, any and all of the causes which have been spoken of as conducive to eczema, in this and other chapters. No single local remedy can be mentioned as of universal value in eczema of the scalp and face, nor is any one internal remedy sufficient from the beginning to the end of any one individual case ; the treatment may require many changes to suit each varying condition. Perhaps the most commonly valuable pre-scription is that of acetate of potassium, nux vomica, and quassia (Formula 2). If there is a tendency to constipa-tion, the mixture of the sulphates (Formula 1), will be of more service, and also especially in acutely developing eczema of this region, It is often well to begin with, and to repeat at certain intervals, a sharp purgative ; and the one to which I have always given the preference from long use, is that frequently referred to, of blue mass, colo-cynth, and ipecac (Formula 13). These pills may be taken two at night and two on the second night following, and if the disease does not yield satisfactorily, this course may be repeated again at the expiration of a week, more or less. If the mixture of the sulphates is not sufficient to keep the bowels in good condition, the pills of aloes and iron (Formula 14) are of the greatest service, and should be taken faithfully and systematically in the man-ner prescribed elsewhere. Where there is a strumous element found, cod-liver oil is not to be forgotten. Ec-

zema in this region requires perhaps more varied and
carefully selected remedies than that of almost any other
portion of the body, and it would be impossible to give all
the indications necessary to guide the practitioner in its
management in every case.   The dyspeptic element so
commonly found in these cases, will at times give the
greatest trouble, but to obtain permanent success with the
eczema a most careful, thorough, and systematic course of
treatment must be entered upon and followed up until the
end is accomplished.   Some of these elements have been
dwelt upon elsewhere, others must be left to the knowledge and judgment of the physician.

If the internal treatment is so important, the local
measures require, if possible, yet greater care and discrimi-
nation in their selection and application.   The first great
principle to be kept in view, as in regard to eczema everywhere, is the avoidance of great irritation, and much that
has been said in the chapter on infantile eczema may be
borne in mind with profit in this connection.   Here almost
more than in eczema of any other region, I am convinced
that errors are most often made in the way of over-stimu-
lation.   The very abundant blood supply of the head,
and the great readiness with which the amount of blood in
the skin here is influenced by exposure to external irritation and also by nervous causes, all combine to call for
protective care in the management of the external integument of these parts.   If stimulants are used it must be
with caution, and alternated with measures of a soothing
character.

One of the most universally serviceable applications
to the scalp is tannin in the form of ointment (Formula
53), although most of the soothing ointments mentioned
in this book may be of value in this condition.   Of almost
more importance than the exact composition of the ointment itself is the manner in which it is applied.   To be

of real service it should be gotten down among the hairs, upon the real seat of the disease ; and to do this great care and patience are generally required. It may here be remarked that it is not necessary to cut the hair for the cure of eczema upon the scalp, although in the case of children it is perhaps preferable to do so in some cases, as the disease can be thus more easily reached. In older persons, also, when the hair is evidently falling rapidly, it may be advisable to cut it, inasmuch as its growth may be thereby stimulated, and by having it shorter the liability to remove it during the treatment of the affected surface is less. But it may be repeated that as a rule, it is not necessary even in the most severe cases of eczema of the scalp, to cut the hair, if the requisite time and patience can and will be employed in making the proper dressing.

It is not my practice, as with many, to have the scalp washed first in order to remove all the crusts before beginning the application, but I generally have the remedy selected used at once, and in a short time the crusts or scales are found to be softened, and the disease modified, so that the washing does not do the harm it otherwise would. The injury done to the raw surface beneath may be so great, if the washing is undertaken at once, as to be an obstacle to the cure of the disease. Whatever ointment or application is decided upon is directed to be freely applied morning and night among the hairs, with as little friction as possible, and yet with a thorough spreading of it by means of the fingers. After from two to four days' application, the scalp may be washed for the first time, although it is occasionally better to allow even a longer period to elapse. This washing may be done either with good old Castile soap, or tar soap ; or, a mixture of the sapo viridis and water in equal parts, or with half the quantity of alcohol (Formula 42), may be used as a shampoo over a basin of water ; or we may employ borax or

carbonate of soda, either of them in the strength of from
four to eight teaspoonfuls to the pint, according to the
amount of grease upon the scalp. An all important
point to be remembered in this connection, is that the
oily applications are to be made again to the scalp at the
earliest possible moment after the washing. That is, the
scalp should be dried with as little friction as possible,
by means of a soft, warm cloth, and the entire diseased
surface gently covered again with the ointment selected,
within as few minutes as possible after the water has left
it, without waiting for the hair to dry. This applies both
to more acute forms of eruption, where protection is
needed against the irritating effects of the atmosphere,
and also to the more chronic forms to be spoken of later;
because in every instance an exudate appears and dries
on the surface, forming an impenetrable coat, through
which the medicament cannot have the entire and proper
action desired. The scalp should not be washed very often.

In eczema of the scalp of younger persons we will find
great benefit from the tar and zinc ointment (Formula 57),
or from a mild white precipitate ointment (Formula 63).
In more chronic, dry, and scaly stages, citrine ointment,
diluted three or more times (Formula 64), is an invalua-
ble agent in removing the disease. When still greater
stimulation is required, the compound tincture of green
soap (Formula 41), may be quickly rubbed upon the part
and followed by a mildly stimulant ointment. In chronic
erythematous and scaly eczema of the scalp, we may obtain great benefit from a lotion of acetate of lead and
castor oil (Formula 44), used freely as a dressing, night
and morning.

Some little care must be exercised in attempting to
restore the growth of the hair after eczema upon the
scalp, for not at all infrequently a new eruption will be
lighted up by stimulating applications given for this pur-

pose. It is well therefore to begin with those which are quite mild and unirritating, and to increase their strength as the skin is found to bear the stimulation. Perhaps the best lotion to begin with is such an one as that containing quinine and bay rum (Formula .45); later such stronger stimulants as those composed of cantharides and capsicum (Formula 46) may be employed.

Erythematous eczema of the face will sometimes long baffle all efforts to give relief to the itching, and applications have to be employed in increasing strength according to the condition of the parts and the effect of the remedies. It is well always to commence with milder preparations, and the tar and zinc ointment (Formula 57), answers best in the main, and if continuously used will generally give great relief. But to be effective any ointment must be kept on the parts all the time, to a greater or less degree; patients will frequently omit it entirely during the day, and even wash the parts thoroughly and leave them in a dry condition. This will often do as much harm to the eruption as can be overcome during the night treatment, and so the case will remain uncured and incurable until other modes of procedure are adopted. The amount of ointment worn during the day need not be great, but the skin must be slightly greased to protect it from the atmosphere, which is harmful to eczematous skins; when the eruption is improving and the greasy condition during the day is peculiarly obnoxious, a lotion may be substituted which contains a little glycerine (Formulæ 31, 35, 38).

In more chronic and rebellious cases the mercurial ointments are of service (Formulæ 59, 62, 65); and as further stimulants we can add frictions with the compound tincture of green soap (Formula 41), or even with caustic potash solutions, beginning first with weak ones, five to ten grains in the ounce. These are all to be fol-

lowed by mild ointments (Formulæ 51, 52, 54), after
being first washed off, if there is much burning. To give
relief to the itching, camphor and chloral may be used,
either alone (Formula 71) or combined with other ointments. The various preparations of tar are of much
service, and may be used in increasing strengths, unless
signs of irritation are developed (Formulæ 58, 60, 65).
But the local treatment of this form will often be extremely unsatisfactory and the closest attention must be
devoted to the general management in order to obtain
success ; for if removed by local measures the eruption
has the strongest tendency to relapse again and again.

Papular and vesicular eczema of the face generally requires mild measures ; when actually developing, dusting
powders are most suitable, such as pure starch or buckwheat flour, alone or combined with astringent remedies
(Formulæ 23, 24, 26). Lotions are also very grateful and
may be freely applied (Formulæ 31, 32, 33) : soothing
ointments may be used at night.

Pustular eczema of the hairy face is often most intractable. Harm is frequently done by harsh applications, but on the other hand mild measures very often
yield but temporary benefit ; very great care is therefore requisite in order that while stimulating sufficiently
undue irritation is not set up. It is almost impossible
to extract the hairs systematically, as is done in sycosis,
the pain is so great, and moreover it is unnecessary and
does not cure the disease. It is generally best to shave
daily if possible, using a very bland soap ; by preference
Pear's English transparent shaving soap. The operation
is painful at first but is soon borne well, and is really necessary in order that the remedies may come into close
contact with the diseased skin, and in order that the stiff
hairs may not further irritate the inflamed surface. Immediately after shaving, the suitable ointment, often the

diachylon (Formula 61), is to be laid on, spread upon lint, and firmly bound on. Some ointment must also be kept applied during the day, though lightly smeared on. If the eruption still resists, stimulation is cautiously added as in eczema elsewhere. Pustular or impetiginous eczema of the non-bearded face is usually a simple affair, and yields readily to continuous application of zinc, or bismuth, or diluted white precipitate ointment, with the avoidance of washing.

Eczema of the eyelids always calls for internal and tonic treatment, and will generally cease with this, combined with very moderate local treatment. The eyes should be soaked by means of a cloth, with hot water in which a little bi-carbonate of soda is dissolved, two to three drachms to the pint. This is done every night, and the edges of the lids are then thoroughly anointed with a diluted red oxide of mercury ointment (Formula 66). Occasionally severe and continued eye strain will be the efficient cause of the eruption on the lids, and this must be rectified; sometimes also errors of accommodation will be at the bottom of the trouble, and properly adjusted glasses will do more for its permanent cure than all other measures.

Eczema about the ears need not generally give difficulty, although these cases often linger for longer periods; the movement of the ear and friction at night, etc., are reasons for the eruption proving obstinate in this locality. When the eruption is severe, the ear must be bound up and thoroughly protected all the time, with a soothing dressing; the ointment should not be rubbed upon the ear but spread upon lint and thoroughly applied to every part. When fresh ointment is replaced, the surface is to be only gently wiped, and all the old ointment need not be gotten off, though if there has been secretion it should be gently cleansed but not washed.

It is not an easy matter to keep the dressings properly applied in this location, and considerable care and ingenuity may be required. Behind the ears especially, the dressings will continually become displaced, and if ointment is simply laid on, it will be all removed by the pillow. The surface behind the ears will often bear stimulation very well, and the compound tincture of green soap (Formula 41), briskly rubbed on and followed by diachylon ointment (Formula 61), thoroughly and continuously applied, will cure many a case which has long exhibited a red and occasionally moist and cracked eczema behind one or both ears.

Eczema of the external auditory canal will sometimes persist for a long time without being recognized, there being only moderate redness, together with considerable scaling, and some itching, both consequent upon the infiltration. For this the ear will be syringed again and again, only to have the canal fill up as before with rather greasy scales. This condition yields, as a rule, completely to tannin ointment, a drachm to the ounce, put thoroughly and deeply in the meatus by means of a camel's hair brush. As in the treatment of eczema elsewhere too much washing does harm, so in eczema of the external auditory canal, too frequent syringing is harmful; every few days, if there is too much accumulation of scales and ointment, it may be syringed out with a little borax or soda and water, and the ointment immediately replaced. If the condition resists this treatment, diluted citrine ointment may be used (Formulæ 64, 65), or the canal may be painted with a weak solution of nitrate of silver (Formula 50.) In the main, however, reliance may be placed upon the faithful use of the tannin ointment or the glycerole of tannin.

CHAPTER XI.

THE same causes which render eczema of the face and scalp rebellious to treatment operate with equal or greater force in regard to eczema of the hands. The eruption in this location is often associated with dyspeptic conditions, and there is reason also to believe 'that reflex nervous influences may operate to cause it more or less potentially: thus, as already mentioned, Hebra asserts that he has known women to have eczema on the hands with each recurring pregnancy, and that such persons could even predict a pregnancy more surely from this sign than from any other. I have known the eruption to recur on the hands with every nervous excitement or depression.

All the possible opportunities of local irritation also exist here even more than on the face. Motion is incessant; scratching is most easily effected; it is difficult to keep remedies perfectly and continuously applied; exposure to air, water, and dust is common. The constant recurrence of the eruption in cooks, laundresses, butlers, and others who put their hands much in water, and the very great difficulty in curing some of these cases while their occupation is continued, illustrate very forcibly the injury from this cause. The exposed position of the parts renders them also peculiarly susceptible to irritation from other external causes, and the dust which continually settles on the hands, and works into the fissures which occur, undoubtedly aggravates the eruption. In addition to the exposures of ordinary life there are others which are incident to occupations, such as those occurring in workers in lime, as masons, plasterers, and brick layers, also in the case of grocers, bakers, and others, where the particles of lime, sugar, flour, etc., and the frequent washings rendered necessary by occupations, all contribute to cause or prolong the eruption ; also workers in dyes and in chemicals, as electro-platers and polishers, are all prone to have rebellious eczema of the hands.

Certain local poisons with which the hands may come in contact must ever be borne in mind, as that of the poison ivy or oak, rhus toxicodendron, and the poison sumach, rhus venenata. Many of the dyes now employed may prove irritating to the skin and I have known a number of instances where the colored lining of gloves has started the eruption ; in several individuals the eruption recurred each time that the gloves were worn. It will be remembered, however, that skin lesions caused by these external irritants alone need not be eczema, but are frequently simply a dermatitis, as before described ; but they may become the starting point for the development of a true eczema if other etiological factors are present.

The manifestations of eczema upon the hands are most varied ; all forms and varieties may occur here, and in addition to those ordinarily observed there are certain other lesions which are well nigh peculiar to the hands, namely, a certain hardening, peeling, and fissuring of the skin of the palms, or the palmar surfaces of the fingers, which may at times involve ends of the fingers alone, without other apparent sign of disease. We may, and not infrequently do, have eczema in the most acute form upon the hands, exhibiting much inflammation, papules, vesicles, and pustules, with considerable œdema. More commonly the disease appears in a sub-acute or chronic form, with the repeated development of papules and vesicles, generally in groups or patches; the affected portion of skin then hardens, becomes infiltrated, may subsequently crack, and we have an even patch of reddened and thickened tissue, itchy and sore, and the source of very great annoyance or even distress. The fissures which form are not always transverse, as one might expect, but often come parallel with the length of the fingers, or diagonally in the palm, and not necessarily in the lines of motion.

The vesicles observed in eczema of the hands are peculiar: when occurring on soft parts as on the back of the hand and sides of the fingers they are small and delicate and rupture quite quickly. But on the ends of the fingers and the palms they are usually very persistent and appear beneath the epidermis as minute spots, slightly darker than the surrounding skin, not at all elevated, but still suggesting of themselves that they contain fluid; and if these are punctured with a needle serum exudes. While the vesicles are unruptured the itching is often very great, but it is largely relieved when the fluid finds exit; patients, therefore, very frequently puncture the vesicles themselves both here and upon the toes, for the thick coating of epidermis retains the fluid a long time unless artificially broken; occasionally we see a number of vesicles running together and stripping up considerable areas of epidermis.

The diagnosis of eczema of the forms just described is not usually a very difficult one, if the features are carefully studied and the elements of eczema well borne in mind. It is well always to exclude scabies first, both because this eruption most closely resembles eczema, and because if scabies remains unrecognized the case cannot be cured. Scabies as is known, generally affects the hands first, and especially the region between the fingers;

and eczema may appear in exactly the same location and
be strongly suggestive of it.   But scabies also affects
other parts at almost the same time, and the signs of the
eruption should be looked for in these places as well:
these other localities liable to be affected in scabies
are, the soft parts about the flexures of the wrist, and
the inner surface of the forearms, the penis in the male
and the neighborhood of the nipple in the female, and
also about the malleoli and the soles of the feet in children.   In eczema, moreover, the papulo-vesicles are apt
to be mostly in groups, whereas in scabies they are more
scattered; in eczema they are more uniform in size, in
scabies they show various grades of inflammation, so that
papules, vesicles, and generally pustules or the remains of
pustules may often be seen at once; the vesicles of eczema usually rupture soon and the surface becomes crusty,
those of scabies remain longer, and on breaking may subside at once or leave a spot of ordinary inflammation.
But the pathognomonic sign of scabies, which when found
is quite sufficient, is the *cuniculus* or furrow made by the
burrowing insect; this is seen as a minute dotted, black
or dirty, curved line, from a tenth to a sixth of an inch in
length, sometimes longer, looking as though a bit of dark
colored sewing silk had been run beneath the skin.
These are usually seen running to and sometimes over a
vesicle or pustule, and the insect is found at the extremity where the inflammation exists.   When vesicles of eczema have ruptured, their margins sometimes present
curved black lines which simulate the cuniculi of scabies,
and some little care may be required to prevent a mistake; the furrows of scabies are unaffected by washing
the part, except to make them more distinct, whereas
the epidermal elevations alluded to almost disappear,
and their true character will be shown in the fringe of
epidermis.   It is not always easy for an inexperienced

person to discover and extract the acarus from the furrow, although if this can be accomplished, the diagnosis is yet more firmly established. There can generally be a history of contagion made out in scabies, although it must be remembered that a whole family may also be affected with eczema simultaneously, without there being any infection.

There are two or three other eruptions which may be confounded with certain cases of eczema of the backs of the hands and fingers. These are lichen planus, erythema papulatum, dysidrosis, and pompholyx or cheiropompholyx. Lichen planus presents always a papular lesion, from first to last, the papules are large, flat on the summit or slightly depressed, with abrupt sides, and thus very different from the sharp, pointed papules of eczema ; their color is of a pinkish purple, and the surface often of a lighter shade, and glazy or shiny. Sometimes the papules run together, forming larger plaques, but there is always an abrupt though slight elevation above the surface, the margins are sharply defined, and there is very little if any scaling. It is a very chronic affection, and the papules may remain almost unchanged for weeks ; there may be considerable itching.

Erythema papulatum is an acute affair characterized by the rather sudden development of quite large, inflammatory papules of various sizes and shapes, often associated with other forms of erythema multiforme, of which it is but one manifestation. There is burning rather than itching, although there may be very little sensation at all, except soreness in the papules ; there is not the tendency to exudation, although some of the lesions may occasionally go on to form large vesicles or bullæ, but when these rupture, the surface heals and there is no infiltration of tissue as in eczema.

Dysidrosis resembles vesicular eczema very closely in

many instances. But it is characterized by deeper seated vesicles, with less inflammatory element than is seen in eczema, and the vesicles have little tendency to break or discharge. The appearance of the watery collections has been likened to boiled sago grains beneath the skin, and after the affection has lasted for a while the epidermis becomes soggy and appears macerated, and there is considerable soreness. Pompholyx or cheiro-pompholyx may have much the same phenomena in its incipiency as dysidrosis, but later on much larger bullæ form, and the disease resembles pemphigus. There is often considerable itching, though the sensation is more commonly that of pricking, burning, or pain.

Eczema of the palms requires special attention because of the difficulties of diagnosis which continually arise, and because accuracy is absolutely essential to successful treatment. The disease may affect little or much of one or both palms, alone or conjoined with the eruption elsewhere. The soles of the feet are affected in a manner almost exactly similar to the palms of the hands, and the present description and differentiation will suffice for both.

The thickness of the epidermis of the palms and soles causes both the lesions to be peculiar and the disease to be obstinate. The lesions of acute eczema are seldom seen on these parts, though with the sub-acute or chronic eruption we continually have the formation of vesicles deep in, giving rise to great itching.

It is the chronic, scaly eczema of the palm and sole which presents the greatest difficulties in diagnosis. The eruption is seen in the form of dry, hard, itchy patches of infiltrated skin, covering a greater or smaller portion of the surface, presenting a moderate, ragged scaling, and generally exhibiting a number of fissures or cracks, which are exceedingly painful. In a severe case the aspect of the hand or foot thus affected is a distressing one. The hand is kept in a half-closed position, the patient fearing to move it, on account of the suffering from the cracks, or from the danger of causing new fissures: the hands are thus often rendered well nigh useless. The feet may be affected in a manner almost precisely similar, but the eruption is apt to be less severe on the soles because of the constant protection of the part and of the continual moisture; the absence of the repeated changes in temperature and moisture to which the hands are subject further explains why the eruption is commonly less severe on the soles than on the palms. Such a lesion as has been described is made infinitely worse by exposure to the air, for the secretion of sweat seems to be almost entirely suspended: when kept constantly wet such hands will be quite flexible, and patients even with a large amount of eruption will sometimes be able to do washing, although each time the hands become dry they are worse, and the after suffering from them may be intense.

The diagnosis of these dry palmar and plantar lesions need not be very difficult if they are closely studied and the following points carefully attended to. There are only three eruptions which can affect the palms and soles in the manner above described; these are syphilis, psoriasis, and eczema. Some recent observers exclude true psoriasis, but there is no doubt that this disease may and does sometimes affect these surfaces as well as all others of the body; of this I have seen several instances. Mr. Wilson states that "eczema squamosum of the palm constitutes one of two forms of psoriasis palmaris which it is important to distinguish, the other being a syphilitic affection." It must be remembered, however, that he applies the term psoriasis not in the sense in which it is now generally used, but to represent only a scaly stage of eczema ; true psoriasis, the lepra of older writers, he calls alphos, and states that he has seen it once or twice on the palms of the hands.

It is so very doubtful as to whether true psoriasis ever affects the palms or soles alone, without appearing elsewhere on the body, notably on the extensor surfaces of the limbs or on the scalp, that it may indeed be stated that it never occurs in these situations alone ; I certainly have never met with it, nor do I know those who have. When seen in this locality it assumes the same form as observed elsewhere, although the appearances are somewhat modified by the very thick, dense, and tough epidermal covering peculiar to the situation. It is in the same round patches, sharply defined and isolated, which increase in size peripherally, and may, of course, if near each other, run together. But there is not the infiltration peculiar to eczema and there is not the same tendency to fissures, though they do occur if a spot happens to be at a flexure of the skin ; but then the fissures are more dry and with less tendency to bleed and to exude ; there is also not the intense itching which generally accompanies eczema until the soreness takes its place.

Psoriasis palmaris is therefore a misnomer for the condition under consideration, although frequently applied to it, and the term is equally inapplicable to the lesion produced by syphilis. The term psoriasis, is at present employed to designate a definite disease affecting the skin, quite distinct from eczema, with whose pathological anatomy we are now well acquainted. True psoriasis of the palms and soles is a very rare disease, and if, as was just stated, it never attacks these parts alone without being present elsewhere, we have at once a very valuable diagnostic mark in dealing with cases of chronic, scaly disease of the palms and soles. We will now consider the only other lesion which may thus affect these parts, namely, an eruption produced by syphilis; this is the papulo-squamous syphiloderm, a scaly papular or tubercular syphilide of the palms and soles, often wrongly called syphilitic psoriasis of these parts.

Syphilis may affect the palms and soles during any period of its existence, but the chronic scaly eruption which may be confounded with eczema in the localities under consideration, is usually seen rather late in the disease, and very frequently exists as the only manifestation of the poison at the time. Early in the course of the malady we may have an acute eruption of many papules on the palms and soles, as a part of a general efflorescence; the diagnosis is then not difficult. A little later, say within two to five years after infection, the eruption is apt to appear symmetrically, affecting both palms or both soles, just as the other lesions of this period are generally symmetrical. Still later on, and this lesion can come as late as twenty years after the primary sore, the eruption may appear upon one palm or sole, and, as remarked before, often constitutes the sole external manifestation of syphilis.

The main point to bear in mind in the differentiation of a syphilitic eruption on the palm or sole from eczema is, that the lesions of syphilis are caused by a new deposit in the skin, attended possibly with secondary signs of inflammation, whereas eczema is an inflammatory affection, and the infiltration is secondary to this. Syphilis of these parts, therefore, begins with the formation of separate papules or tubercles; often a single one will be first noticed, and the new accessions are marked, not by a gradual extension of the diseased surface, but by the appearance of additional papules or tubercles on or near the margin. Eczema, on the other hand, while it may begin at a single point, which is not very common, extends peripherally by the spreading of the inflammatory process, and not by the accession of new elements.

When either affection has lasted some time, many of the sharp differential marks are lost, and if attention is paid only to the central portions, or those most affected, the diagnosis will be almost impossible, for both may present an evenly reddened surface, bereft of healthy epidermis, perhaps exhibiting painful fissures, and with a ragged border of unhealthy epidermis. But generally, if not always, a careful study of the patch, and especially of the margins, will detect points which will serve to establish the true character of the eruption.

Remembering the pathological conditions before mentioned, we will generally find at or outside of the border of the fully diseased surface, if the lesion be syphilitic, one or many small, well defined, hard papules over which the epidermis has broken more or less. It will be recognized that the death of the epidermis and its exfoliation in the syphilitic manifestation is a secondary matter, owing to the interference with its nutrition by the presence of the new deposit beneath; whereas the epidermal destruction in an eczematous eruption, is a part of the disease process, here as elsewhere.

At or near the margin of an eczema of the palm or sole, on the other hand, will generally be observed some lesions which are characteristic of this eruption, namely; deep vesicles, or inflammatory papules, or erythema, and, as previously remarked, eczema of the palms or soles is usually not the only manifestation of the disease.

The differences between the syphilitic and eczematous eruption on the palms or soles is also seen by a careful examination of the margin or border of the affected patches. In syphilis, the lesions which have been spoken of as characteristic will generally be seen: that is, the border of a patch of syphilitic eruption will be found to be scalloped and uneven, for the reason that it has been formed by the fresh development and union of many small papulo-tubercles. For the same reason the epidermis is raised on the margin towards the centre of the eruption, and when pulled on or stripped back it is found to run down into healthy skin, and cannot be torn off without causing pain. The margin of an eczema patch is less sharply defined, but fades more into healthy skin, or, if there is a punched out epidermal edge there is erythematous redness beyond it. The margin of the eczematous patch also does not present the uneven aspect of the syphilitic one, but is in larger curves.

When eczema has passed over a surface it leaves the skin in a thickened condition, which persists, and the centre of all eczema patches are, as a rule, as bad as or worse than the edges. With syphilis of the palm or sole there is a tendency for the portion which has been traversed by the disease to heal, so that we frequently see only a margin of eruption, in which separate papules or tubercles can be clearly made out, and a reddened surface behind with imperfectly formed epidermis, but without the thickening or infiltration and cracks belonging to eczema. Frequently, however, new masses will form on the portions previously affected by syphilis, and these, equally with the masses on the edge, may present ugly and painful fissures.

The itching accompanying eczema of the palm or sole is generally very severe, and adds greatly to the distress occasioned by the cracks : in syphilis there is little if any itching, and the cracks are not apt to be so abundant, they may generally be seen to be across a papule, whereas the fissures of eczema occur anywhere, independently of any special localized infiltration, and often quite independent of the lines of flexion of the hands.

The eruption of syphilis seldom extends on to the

backs of the fingers or hands, whereas very commonly eczema in this region will creep around, and present ordinary characters in this location. The syphiloderm may, however, extend to a moderate degree around either side of the hand, and even occupy the sides of the fingers when the eruption is very extensive as is sometimes the case, it covering all the palmar surface of the hands and fingers.

In certain rare instances we have both a true eczema of the palmar or plantar surface and a syphilitic eruption combined with it. These cases are very difficult of accurate diagnosis and yet more difficult to treat. But a little care will demonstrate the points described as syphilitic, while an eczema element existing here or elsewhere will show the features of this eruption. In these instances a combined treatment is necessary, both that which will be shortly detailed for the eczema and that appropriate for the syphilitic lesion. But while the simple, uncomplicated syphilitic cases yield with marvellous rapidity, and most of the eczematous lesions also can be managed satisfactorily, these complex cases resist remedial measures most annoyingly.

There is another form or manner in which eczema sometimes affects the palms which is quite different from that just described, and which would be very difficult of recognition if it were not previously understood. The entire surface may be evenly attacked, and there results a thickened, hard, and rather glazy surface, with little or no scaling, but accompanied with considerable itching, and a stiffness which almost incapacitates the hand for work; there may also occur fissures, although they are not apt to be so deep as when the eruption is more localized, as in the condition previously described. This state is very much like that ordinarily obtained in the palms of those accustomed to much hard, manual work; but these cases differ from this ordinary callosity in the diffuse character of the lesion, in the itching and cracking, and in occurring often in those who seldom if ever use the hands for physical labor.

A condition similar to that just described is frequently seen upon the ends of the fingers alone, and presents a state which would not ordinarily be recognized as eczema, certainly not by those who look for vesicles or even papules as necessary lesions of this eruption. This consists of a dry, hard state of the skin, with fissures and more or less peeling of the hardened epidermis. There is but little itching usually accompanying it, but there is generally a very considerable degree of discomfort from the stiffness and from the roughened epidermis, which catches in articles of clothing, especially in woolens; and often much pain from the cracks which may sometimes be deep. The nails are not usually affected in this connection, although sometimes the nail bed at the free extremity becomes thickened and the nail itself is attacked, being thickened, brittle, and stubbed. There is no eruption with which this dry, hard eczema of the tips of the fingers can be confounded ; the condition of the nails just described however, is very much like that seen in parasitic disease of the nail. But in parasitic nail disease, which is rare, there is often a vegetable parasitic eruption present elsewhere, or there is a history of exposure, perhaps in treating or having close relations with some one affected with ringworm or favus.

Eczema of the nails, nail-beds, and furrows around the nails is not of very uncommon occurrence, either alone or associated with the eruption elsewhere. It is an annoying affection, and sometimes very obstinate. The fold of skin around the base of the nail will be found thickened and red, with abraded points upon it, which may exude if irritated, and the whole surface is generally very itchy. If it has been of long duration, especially at the base of the nail, the nail itself will be found affected ; it will have lost its smoothness and appears rough, misshapen and uneven on the surface, sometimes marked by transverse and sometimes by longitudinal furrows, often with minute depressions or holes over its surface, and near the root it is very likely to be much depressed. In an acute attack the nail may be shed more or less completely. In more chronic states it becomes brittle, and either thickened at its free extremity or greatly thinned, and in either case it will chip off with each attempt to use the fingers, as in buttoning the clothes, etc. If the furrows at the sides of the nails are mainly affected, the nail may escape much or any distortion. As the disease is arrested, the healthy nail grows more and more evenly from its root, and may sometimes regain almost a normal appearance, while some eczema elements are still present at the base and sides of the nail. Even very badly disfigured nails will become quite normal under carefully directed treatment, although in very long standing cases the habit of wrong growth seems to be acquired, and the nails continue misformed even after the eczema has been removed.

Eczema of the arms does not present any features worthy of special diagnostic mention. In the flexure of the elbows it takes the form of acute, sub-acute, or chronic, more or less moist, itchy, red surfaces, which may become so much affected that free motion of the limbs is impossible, because of the cracks which form. But the eruption in this locality is not as frequent as is generally supposed, indeed in my experience it is seen here comparatively rarely. Eczema of the rest of the arms is very generally papular, the papules being either scattered or grouped together in patches of various sizes ; the arms are seldom affected alone, but generally in conjunction with eczema of other parts.

The prognosis of eczema of the hands, as may be judged from what has been said in regard to its etiology, is not so favorable as is that of some other portions of the

body. Even where all proper attention can be paid to
them, external irritants avoided, and the dressings kept
applied as directed, the eruption will sometimes prove
quite rebellious to treatment ; but if all the necessary pre-
cautions are observed, the eruption may certainly be
cured in this locality as well as in any other, although
more time may be required, and the eruption is prone to
relapse from the many causes which excited it. Where
the eruption depends upon the occupation, and this cannot be altered, a perfect and permanent cure may not be
possible ; but even in these cases very much may be done
to alleviate the pain or annoyance caused by it, and the
vocation may even be pursued with comfort, which before
was impossible or extremely distressing.

In regard to the treatment of eczema of the hands,
I will speak mainly of the local measures to be employed, inasmuch as the internal treatment and general
management does not differ greatly from that called for
in eczema of other regions. But as stated at the beginning of the chapter, especial attention must be paid to
the digestive organs, whether they appear affected or
not on casual inquiry, because eczema of the hands is
constantly found to be closely associated with dyspeptic
and nervous conditions.

Acute inflammatory eczema of the hands, owing to
distinct exciting causes, should not give much difficulty
in treatment. To a certain extent it is a self-limited
affection which rapidly improves under a removal of the
cause, together with soothing treatment. Dusting powders (Formulæ 23, 24), or simple flour or powdered starch,
or buckwheat flour, answer very well if there is not much
or any discharge ; these should be kept on the parts all the
time, and this may be conveniently accomplished by keeping the hands in loose bags of muslin, within which a certain amount of the powder is placed, which then applies

itself with every movement of the hands. In highly inflamed states, it is of service to keep the parts continually covered with a soothing and astringent lotion containing a powder, which is deposited upon the skin (Formulæ 31, 32). Or the part may be wrapped in a single fold of muslin, which is kept continually wet with the lead and opium wash (Formula 39). If there is much itching or discharge, a little carbolic acid may be added to the lotion, with advantage. Lotions, however, cannot be advantageously used at night, as the cloth will dry and adhere to the skin, whereas if it is covered with an impermeable dressing, as oiled silk, to prevent evaporation, a poultice is formed and the parts are soddened and relaxed. Ointments therefore will be of more service at night, and that of zinc half a drachm to the ounce, spread thickly upon prepared lint, is the most suitable. On removing it in the morning it is not well to attempt to wash the part too much, but simply to wipe it gently with old muslin or linen, and immediately to reapply the lotion. Diachylon ointment (Formula 61) is used by many in acute eczema, but even when prepared properly, I have not found it as valuable in this state as other remedies ; it is frequently too heating to the part.

Sub-acute and chronic eczema of the backs of the hands and knuckles, will sometimes prove most rebellious, and while soothing measures are of temporary benefit, they are generally incapable of entirely removing the disease, and stimulants have to be resorted to. Eczema in this situation is usually attended with very great itching, and for a mildly stimulating ointment to meet this indication, that composed of zinc and tar (Formula 57), is most valuable. To be of much service it should be kept continually bound on, night and day, spread thickly on the prepared lint, and changed once or twice in the twenty-four hours. With proper constitutional and general management, this will often be sufficient to cure the case, if persisted in; but generally some additional stimulant must be added from time to time.

In regard to the application of stimulant measures, it is to be remembered, as stated in the chapter on general treatment, that the end sought for is not the immediate healing of the part by the stimulating remedy, but, on the other hand, the design is to remove imperfectly formed elements and to excite chronically inflamed tissues to activity, and that a result of this activity may even be an acute form of the eruption. But it must also be remembered that time is to be given for the acute condition to subside under proper soothing treatment, otherwise prolonged and repeated stimulation results in irritation, not very different from that which excited the eruption. The compound tincture of green soap (Formula 41), is recommended by many in the treatment of this condition, and sometimes is of value. But I prefer, as a rule, to use caustic potash in solution, varying in strength from five to ten, twenty or more grains to the ounce; this is quickly rubbed on for a few minutes, and rinsed off with cold water, and the part pretty quickly dried; the ointment which should be previously made ready, spread on lint, is now thoroughly and firmly applied.

As an instance of the value of severe stimulating measures in certain cases, I may mention that of a plasterer whom I treated sometime since with eczema of the backs of the hands: there was a very great thickening of the entire surface, and also of the backs of the fingers. As he was out of work for some time I gave him very severe scrubbings with, I believe, a twenty grain solution of caustic potash; there was of course very considerable reaction from it and he complained a good deal of the pain. Later on I had him employ frictions with common domestic soft soap and an ordinary scrubbing brush. This of course denuded the surface a great deal, but still he scrubbed bravely, resting the hand on a table, the surface being afterwards treated with diachylon ointment, and part of the time with pure mutton tallow. This patient has been repeatedly under my care since that time, now nearly eleven years ago, but although he has eczema of the sides of the fingers and elsewhere, from the plaster, still I have always remarked that the seat of · the original main trouble, the backs of the hands, remained free, being soft and supple. But it must also be remembered that this stimulating treatment may sometimes be followed by very considerable and even troublesome acute inflammation, as in the case cited toward the close of the chapter on general treatment, and it should therefore be advised with caution and the results carefully watched.

Localized patches of eczema of the backs of the hands and fingers, can sometimes be very efficiently removed by blistering ; but I have seen the disease resist most severe and even repeated vesication. Sometimes, indeed, it is very difficult to raise a blister by cantharides upon a patch of chronic eczema.

Eczema in and about the nails, is to be treated in somewhat the same manner, by frictions with caustic potash solutions, and the subsequent envelopment in an astringent ointment. For this purpose the diachylon (Formula 61), serves very well, or an ointment of the persulphate of iron (Formula 67), will sometimes suffice when all else fails. An important addition to the treatment of eczema of the ends of the fingers, and about the nails, is the use of hot water. To obtain the best results from it, it should be used very hot, so hot indeed that the fingers can be put in it but a very short length of time. They are then immersed again for a few seconds, and this is repeated for a not longer period than two or three minutes altogether, and the part is immediately dried and enveloped in one of the ointments mentioned. I have frequently had good results from touching the cracks of eczema about the hands and fingers with a stick of nitrate of silver; this gives considerable pain for the moment, but is generally followed by rapid healing of the particular crack. Sometimes however, this seems to do harm, and the cracks heal slowly after it, and with much pain.

Eczema of the palms and soles, may at times prove very rebellious indeed to treatment, local measures seeming to have very little effect, although in other cases very rapid results are obtained by means of proper local measures. Great benefit can be derived from the use of hot water in this condition, employed in the manner just described in connection with eczema of the ends of the fingers. The palms are laid upon the surface of a basin of very hot water, which is so hot that the hand cannot be thrust wholly into it. After thus touching the palm to the surface, and holding it there for some seconds, it is withdrawn and the contact is repeated several times, but not altogether longer than two or three minutes; the part is then dried, and the ointment which has been previously spread upon lint, cut of a shape to fit the parts, is quickly laid upon it, and bound firmly on. The diachylon ointment generally serves the best for this purpose, and should be continuously applied. Also an ointment containing the liquor picis alkalinus (Formula 62), is of value; likewise one containing calomel (Formula 68). I have had also very good results from the repeated rubbing into the palms of the oleate of mercury, in a five or ten per cent solution. When the eruption resists these measures, stronger stimulation may be resorted to, and for this purpose active scrubbing with the green soap alone or in a solution (Formula 42), may be employed, followed by one of the ointments mentioned; also caustic potash solutions of a strength varying from ten to thirty grains to the ounce, according to the case. In each instance the application is to be washed off, and followed by a suitable ointment. Where there is a considerable accumulation of epidermis, hard and resisting, it is useful to remove this by means of pumice stone, before the application of the ointment.

As this condition progresses towards cure, milder measures may be employed, and the thorough and repeated application to the hands of a lotion containing the glycerole of the sub-acetate of lead (Formula 37), will often prove of the greatest service. This is also of value in lighter forms of eczema of the palm and eczema of the backs of the hands or fingers; it is to be not only thoroughly rubbed in, morning and night, but also one or more times during the day, certainly after every washing of the hands, which should occur as seldom as possible.

Rubber gloves may also be used to very great advantage in many cases of eczema of the hands. To obtain the best results from them they should be worn day as well as night; but this is often very difficult to insure, for patients soon weary of the annoyance of having the hands continually enveloped in a dressing which is both clumsy and uncomfortable. As ordinarily obtained, the rubber gloves have a woven lining of cotton stuff, although certain gloves are in the market made of the pure rubber; but these latter are exceedingly fragile and cannot be depended upon. To obviate the irritating effect from the friction of the cloth lining next to eczematous surfaces, which is heightened by its absorption and retention of the exudation from the diseased parts, I have directed patients using them to turn them directly inside out, buying for this purpose a left hand glove when the right hand was affected, and *vice versa.* By this means we obtain a surface of pure rubber next to the skin, while externally we have the cloth which better resists the wear and tear which generally destroys rubber gloves very quickly if worn in the ordinary manner: the destruction being aided by the separation of the lining from the rubber by means of the moisture within, aided by the greasy matter remaining from ointments.

Many cases of eczema of the hands may be treated locally by this means alone, together with proper constitutional management. The gloves should be drawn off occasionally and allowed to air once or twice a day; for cleansing, the glove should be rinsed out morning and night and left exposed for half an hour to the air. Eczema about the ends of the fingers and nails may be often treated advantageously by means of pure rubber caps, or finger ends. But as ordinarily employed, these are seldom worn for a sufficient length of time to make the cure permanent.

Eczema upon the forearms and arms does not usually present much difficulty in the way of management. At the bend of the elbow it will usually yield quite readily to reasonably mild applications, such as the ointment of zinc and tar (Formula 57), kept closely applied; the addition of the compound tincture of green soap well rubbed upon the part, in the manner directed elsewhere, followed by an ointment, will suffice to remove any thickening which remains. If still greater stimulation is needed one of the mercurial ointments (Formulæ 62–68), will be of service, but the skin on the arms is rather delicate and care must be taken not to overstimulate. Where much of the surface of the arm is affected, and, as is usually the case, there is also an eruption upon other parts, the condition will be best treated by means of baths, which will be described more particularly in the chapter devoted to eczema of the trunk, and general eczema. When the eruption is dry and papular, very great relief may be obtained by rubbing in with the hand a powder, containing chloral and camphor (Formula 25), or by an inunction with an oil containing a tarry preparation (Formula 49).

The eczematous inflammation which sometimes occurs around and in connection with vaccination is generally of a very acute type and requires very delicate handling. Here protection is best afforded by the free application, upon lint, of the oxide of zinc or bismuth ointment half a drachm to the ounce, and it is well to add a little carbolic acid, five or ten grains to the ounce, inasmuch as there is apt to be considerable suppuration present. Care must be taken not to tear off the dressing harshly if it becomes adherent to the surface ; if it is necessary to remove it the mass should be softened by water dressings or by soaking with almond or cod liver oil. It is often far better, however, to leave on the portion which adheres to the sore, cutting off the rest, and dressing the whole again, with the protective ointment. Of late there has been a vaccination protective shield offered for sale, which I have found of great service in preventing this part from being rubbed by the clothing. It consists in a framework of wire, suitably protected, which is attached to the arm by means of tapes: beneath this the dressings rest undisturbed, and a great amount of suffering and annoyance may be saved by this simple device, if properly adjusted.

degree to the defective circulation belonging to this region. Not only is this portion of the body farthest removed from the centre of circulation, but the dependent posture usually assumed augments the difficulty, which is often further increased by the binding of garters or tightly fitting stockings and underclothes.

The exposed position of the legs, and their liability to injury and also to the effects of cold, render the skin in this region peculiarly susceptible to eczema, and also to the formation of ulcers.

Eczema of the legs may exhibit all the phases of the eruption shown elsewhere, but it most commonly takes the form known as *eczema rubrum or madidans*. When fully developed this is characterized by a raw, red, moist, weeping or "leeting" surface, accompanied with much burning pain and aching, or jtching when the skin becomes dry. But the eruption is not always present in its most characteristic form, and often the applicability of the name cczema rubrum is not at once apparent; for, when first seen the limb may be more or less covered with large yellowish and brownish scales or crusts, sometimes of considerable size, and only between the cracks in these can any red surface or moisture be seen. But these crusts or scales are found to be easily detached, and beneath them there is a slightly moist, reddened condition of skin, and if a water dressing or an impermeable covering be applied, there results a surface bereft of normal epidermis, reddened, and exuding a sticky fluid. If now this be kept covered with dressings which exclude the air, or if it be frequently cleansed, it remains red and moist, discharging a greater or less quantity of this sticky, glairy secretion. If it is left exposed to the air it dries, and there are again formed the same scaly and crusted masses.

The extent and severity of eczema on the legs will vary very greatly in different individuals, from a single patch of erythematous or papular eruption of small size, to one covering both limbs entirely, and giving the greatest amount of suffering. The progress is sometimes very rapid, and what appears as a rather insignificant spot of erythematous eczema may spread in a few days so as to cover the limb; although in another case a patch will remain quiescent for a long time. There is considerable deep, aching pain connected with eczema of the lower extremities, and often the evidence of an extension of the disease will be manifested by a pain and tenderness on pressure beyond the line of eruption.

Thus far, diffuse, erythematous eczema, breaking down with an exuding surface has only been mentioned. Other forms are also seen, though less commonly, on the lower leg; we may have chronic patches, with hard, infiltrated skin, and great itching, or, a more or less generalized, papular eruption, with exuding points when scratched. But these forms are far more frequently associated with eczema of other parts, whereas the condition first described is frequently the sole manifestation of the disease. Typical eczema rubrum is rarely seen in children or young persons, but usually occurs after thirty years of age, more commonly even after forty.   In younger persons eczema of the legs is almost invariably associated with eczema elsewhere, and may assume a vesicular or pustular character.

Eczema of the legs should not present much difficulty in diagnosis.   There are very few conditions which could be mistaken for that described, but two indeed ever greatly resemble it, namely erysipelas and psoriasis.   Many of these cases of erythematous eczema, are wrongly called " erysipelas," but, as stated in connection with eczema of the face, it is to be remembered that erysipelas is an acute affection, with constitutional symptoms, and presents very different local phenomena from those here described ; moreover, it does not exist as a chronic disease.   Psoriasis also exhibits very different features, with its separate, well-defined, scaly patches, generally round ; it also generally exists elsewhere in a characteristic appearance.   When the eruption of eczema has become scaly, it is often called psoriasis ; but this is a misnomer, the two are distinct affections and eczema does not become psoriasis when it assumes a scaly phase.

Very commonly eczema of the lower legs is associated with varicose veins to a greater or less degree ; these may be large and tortuous, but they are also quite as frequently deep seated, and are only discoverable on passing the finger over the limb with a little pressure.   When present in this deep, slightly-marked form, small soft depressions, with hard edges, will mark the seat of the thickened and dilated veins, with their valves rendered almost useless by disease ; these are quite as important indications as are the large veins which are visible.   In other cases the weakened state of the blood vessels is seen in a dilatation of the capillaries of the foot.   In yet other cases the impeded circulation may exhibit very few of the signs ordinarily recognized, and yet the eczema may be largely the result of the weakened state of the blood vessels, and will be benefited by the same measures as are of service in the well marked varicose state.

The varicose ulcer is a very common accompaniment or complication of eczema of the lower leg, and indeed is but a heightened condition or state of the same eczematous process, and this tendency of the tissues to break down will often render the eczema very rebellious to treatment; although in the rubber bandage, to be described later, we have almost a specific for these ulcers and also for eczema of this region.

The diagnosis of varicose ulceration presents, in the main, the single difficulty of differentiation from syphilitic ulceration ; this must always be carefully made, otherwise the measures to be described will be useless. Ulcers of syphilitic origin are rarely found on the lower portion of the limb alone, without the existence of present or previous ulceration above the middle line, or even on the upper third of the leg ; thus, about the knee there will not infrequently be seen scars of previous lesions. Generally the syphilitic ulcer, which is the result of a broken down tubercular or gummy deposit, has a sharply cut edge, slightly undermined, and a greyish, pultaceous floor, and the pus, which is abundant, is exceedingly fetid ; the points of ulceration also are numerous and are rather more apt to be located around or toward the back or fleshy part of the calf, whereas varicose ulcers and those from eczema are generally seen toward the front. The edges of the latter are hard, brawny, and everted, and the secretion is not abundant nor fetid, but they are inclined to bleed easily, and are very painful as the dressings are removed. When the ulcers of syphilis have lasted a long time, however, they are very apt to take on the individual characters of the non-specific ulceration; but generally their location, number, and tendency to circular shape or disposition will make the diagnosis plain , especially if there is an absence of varicose veins, and if there exist any scars of preceding ulceration : for further details consult page 61.

Eczema is very prone to attack the popliteal spaces in young persons, less commonly so in adults ; here it presents the ordinary characteristics of a more or less evenly reddened and thickened surface, often quite papular, with marks of scratching, and' perhaps with some moderate scaling or crusting. When severe, fissures or cracks may form and walking may be rendered very painful. Generally, however, the eruption in this location gives its principal annoyance by the itching, which at times is very severe indeed.

Eczema of the thighs is generally conjoined with eczema of other parts. It may assume the erythematous or the papular form ; vesicles and moist surfaces of any extent are seldom seen here, though acute eczema may form large patches on these parts. The itching is often excessive, and a large share of· the lesions will often be the direct result of scratching. The eruption seen about the fork of the thighs and genital region, which has been known as eczema marginatum, the tinea trichophytina cruris or ringworm of these parts, often very closely resembles ordinary eczema ; this will be found fully described in connection with the management of eczema of the anus and genital region.

There is an affection with which eczema of the thighs and legs is often confounded and which it may sometimes resemble quite closely : this is true prurigo. First it may be stated that this disease is an exceedingly rare one in the United States, not over two or three undoubted cases having been thus far observed and recorded by those occupied with this branch. The chances are, therefore, infinitely against any particular case being this eruption. The papules of prurigo are hard and shotty, and often of the color of the skin until scratched ; they are often rather felt than seen. The glands in the groin may sometimes swell in chronic eczema as in prurigo. Pruritus hiemalis is sometimes mistaken for eczema, but here the itching is the chief symptom, and the lesions appear only as the result of scratching; and moreover, these artificial, torn points heal very quickly and there is not any tendency to form patches or exuding surfaces.

Upon the ankles eczema will sometimes prove most seriously obstinate, and the most patient endeavors at its removal will occasionally prove ineffectual for weeks or even months. Here it is generally seen in the form of hard and thickened patches, composed of papules crowded together, of a dark red color, intensely itchy, and inclined to be dry and covered with a horny epidermis, unless scratched or altered by treatment. The eruption is also frequently situated upon the instep and gives rise to great annoyance.

Eczema may affect the foot acutely, although this is rare, except in connection with acute, more or less general eczema, and even then sometimes the feet are spared. It may linger about and between the toes in a sub-acute condition, and thus give rise to much inconvenience. Eczema also attacks the nails of the feet in a manner similar to that described in reference to the nails of the hands.

When the soles of the feet are affected with eczema there may be considerable difficulty in diagnosis if the disease exists there alone, which, however, is rarely the case. The features presented, and the differential diagnosis of the eruption from other lesions are the same as dwelt on in connection with eczema of the palms, and need not be repeated here.

The constitutional or general treatment of eczema of the lower extremities does not differ in principle from that belonging to the disease elsewhere. But there is special necessity that care be paid to the action of the bowels, for the clinical observation may be made daily that the eruption in these cases is always vastly worse whenever constipation occurs, and obstructed portal circulation undoubtedly has a great influence in the production and continuance of the eruption. If possible, this element is even more important when the lower extremities are affected than when the disease is situated in the anal and genital region, where, as will appear in the succeeding chapter, it forms a most prominent feature in the causation of the eruption, under which head it will be fully discussed. The condition of the urine should also receive most careful attention, for not at all infrequently there is deficiency of renal action in eczema rubrum of the lower extremities.

Occasionally eczema of the legs will be one of the first indications of a general break down, especially in persons past forty or forty-five years of age, and indeed a severe eczema of the lower extremities may always be taken as a sign of very greatly impaired health and nutrition, and the most active tonics may be required; eczema in this location should always lead to careful investigation of the general health and should never be neglected or treated with purely local or palliative measures.

There is no doubt but that a varicose condition of the veins is a very large element of causation in many of these cases, as previously alluded to, and it is also true that occupations which compel one to be on the feet very greatly conduce to develop both the varicosity and the eczema. But the same line of argument holds true here which was given in connection with the subject of the causation of eczema in other localities. The local predisposing cause is not alone sufficient of itself, for of the multitudes whose occupation requires their standing very many hours during the day, comparatively few have varicose veins, and of these latter a still smaller number develop

eczema : and again one sees many cases of eczema where
no varicose veins can be made out.   Other causes exist,
and careful and complete medical investigation will seldom
fail to detect impairment of health and of function, and,
as remarked before, abdominal disorder can generally be
demonstrated ; portal congestion, and hepatic and renal
inactivity as a rule exist in these cases.

But the local, exciting causes must also be recognized,
for they furnish the starting point of the eruption ; such
are, bruises and abrasions, the irritation of woolen drawers,
and sometimes poisonous dyes, more commonly in socks.
But a still more potent local exciting cause is found in
scratching, which must ever be borne in mind for it plays
a very important part in the production and continuance
of the eruption.   There is often a little itching in the
limb, and the patient gives way repeatedly to the desire
to scratch, until, from an apparently healthy skin there
may result a large raw surface, or an ulceration of some
size ; and if this is scratched and torn it will not heal, but
remains and increases indefinitely.

The erect posture was spoken of as a cause of the varicose veins and of the eczema, but it is to be noticed that it
is not alone the weight of the increased column of blood
which causes this venous disturbance, but that another
element comes in, which is of great importance to remember from a therapeutical standpoint.   It is to be remarked
that the patients with varicose veins, ulcers, and eczema
of the lower leg are not those who are on their feet in
walking, but these conditions are found in those who are
obliged to stand for a considerable length of time, if not all
day, more or less quiet.   Thus, one rarely sees these troubles in post-carriers, who walk from ten to twenty or more
miles daily, nor even in policemen, who walk about when
on duty, many hours each day ; but it is found among
those with such occupations as cooks, laundresses, type

setters, car drivers, wood-turners, and others who remain long standing without much active movement.

A little consideration of the mechanism of the circulation will explain the difference. The impulse of the blood from the heart is sufficient to carry it to the utmost parts of the body and to force it into every available opening. As it approaches the periphery the circulatory system expands more and more, until from the single aorta there results an infinity of capillaries, whose total area is enormous, and the current of blood in them is proportionately slowed and impeded. These are now gathered into the veins and a comparatively sluggish stream is returned to the heart. Under ordinary circumstances this *vis a tergo* is quite sufficient to return the blood properly, as is seen in sleep, where the process proceeds with regularity and perfection.

But there is another element in the circulation which is of vital importance, especially as relates to the lower extremities. It is well known that the veins have valves directed towards the heart, which are especially large in the vessels of the lower extremities. These are of more service than simply to prevent the blood from returning when it has welled up from the capillaries. They are active elements of the circulation, they are indeed the valves belonging to a second, heart-like power which assists in propelling the blood, namely the voluntary muscles of the limbs and trunk. Each time that the muscle contracts, as in walking, the blood is forced from it, and from the flaccid veins which it surrounds, and as it cannot be crowded backward because of the valves in the veins, the current is forced onward towards the heart. Now when there is not the alternate contraction and relaxation of the muscles from constant use, but simply a constant strain, as in standing, the circulation loses just this impulse, and the veins, unable to stand the constant pressure unaided, become dilated, the valves are stretched open and cease to act, and all the consequences of the impeded circulation result.

Further, with this slowed and imperfect venous current there naturally follows a defective and blocked capillary circulation, and as a consequence a retarded absorption of the waste products from the tissues, and hence the tedious removal of the results of inflammation, eczematous and other. With this incomplete capillary action the lymphatics find the performance of their functions interfered with; the same causes which produce a sluggish venous circulation operate also to retard that of the lymphatics; they become blocked, and in long standing cases the glands at the groin and elsewhere become enlarged, and they cannot even do their own proper work. The part which simple debility can play in the production and continuance of disease on the lower extremities can also be readily understood. Lessened heart power involves imperfect capillary circulation, also weakened muscular action, and relaxed capillaries. Exudation from them is thereby favored, and absorption of effused products hindered.

The therapeutic importance of this study relates to affording proper support for the limb affected with eczema or varicose ulceration. Happily in the rubber bandage we have a measure which has almost revolutionized the management of this class of troubles, and which has cured and can cure many cases which formerly were most intractable, if indeed they were not practically incurable.

The principle of support to the limb has long been recognized, and various methods have been employed to effect this result, in the way of roller bandages of different materials, elastic and laced stockings, etc. But very considerable experience, first in the employment of other measures, and for the last five years in the very extensive use of the solid rubber bandage, leads me to say most decidedly that in the vast majority of cases the solid rubber bandage is unexcelled for the management of eczema, and also of eczematous and varicose ulcers of the lower extremities. This judgment is formed not only from the good results observed daily by means of it, but also from a careful comparison of these cases with those where other means were employed. And this not only from my own practice, but from observing cases in the hands of others.

The rubber bandage yields with every motion of the limb, as the cotton or flannel bandage cannot, and by its constant, elastic pressure supplies what is lost of the natural elasticity of the skin by disease. Even if rubber or any impervious dressing is placed beneath an ordinary roller bandage, in order to obtain the results of maceration, upon which some would explain the efficacy of the rubber bandage, we have still the unyielding character of the envelopment, as contrasting strongly with the generously elastic nature of that made of pure, solid rubber. If the rubber bandage cannot be obtained, one of flannel (with something beneath to protect the parts), is better than one of cotton or linen ; or, still better, are the elastic, open, linen bandages recently made in England.

As contrasted with the elastic stockings formerly employed, the rubber bandage has very great superiority. While the former is of a definite, fixed size, and even stretches with age, thus becoming looser as the limb becomes smaller, the rubber bandage is adapted to the daily requirements of the part, and may be applied loosely if there should chance to be more swelling, while as the limb grows smaller under treatment the bandage follows it, and may be made to suit the necessities of the case to the very end. Moreover, the process of application and removal of the elastic stocking may give much irritation to the diseased surfaces, both by the manipulations necessary and by the rough, uneven, and often irritating char-

acter of the stocking, and its tendency to adhere to the
affected parts.   The solid rubber bandage leaves a moist
surface, and on its removal no violence is done to the tender, newly-formed tissues beneath.   In regard to the relative expense, the rubber bandages are very much cheaper,
while under proper care they will outlast the stocking; I
have known the same bandage to be worn continuously
for from six months to a year.   In regard to using bandages made of a woven, elastic, rubber webbing, such as is
often used in securing bloodless operations by Esmarch's
method, I have no experience whatever.   This material
could be employed, but would require something beneath
it to protect both the diseased surface and the bandage,
and the smooth, non-irritating surface of the pure rubber
could hardly be replaced by any other with advantage;
moreover, the gain from the maceration obtained with the
pure rubber would be lost.

The hard, unyielding laced stocking cannot be compared with the rubber bandage for utility and comfort; it
combines the disadvantages of the ordinary cotton bandage, and those of the elastic stocking.

A few words may be added in regard to the details
necessary for the successful use of the rubber bandage.
First, as to the cases in which it may be employed.

It may be applied with success even to eczema presenting very acute phenomena, although, as a rule, acutely
developing cases do not bear it so well.   When first put
on the patient may shrink from the application of the
rubber directly to a diseased part, but it will generally be
found to be not only well borne, but of great comfort to
the sufferer.

The rubber bandage, however, is especially serviceable
in the more chronic cases, such as usually resist all measures commonly employed.   In these cases where there is
a long standing, red, very itchy, and scaly condition of

skin covering a larger or smaller portion of the limb, it may be applied at once, and with the expectation of the greatest relief. The bandage may and often does cause an eruption of its own for a short time, sometimes for a longer period; this takes the form of a few scattered, minute, superficial pustules, running their course rapidly. But these need not interfere with its employment, as they soon cease to be produced, and the affected surface heals kindly. Occasionally it may be best to place a cotton bandage or piece of thin linen well fitted, beneath the rubber bandage; but as a rule this is not required, and far more frequently it does harm instead of good.

The bandage is particularly serviceable, as before stated, in those cases where ulceration exists; and especially in those which are associated with enlarged or varicose veins. In many of these cases it forms the sole treatment, and is alone sufficient for a perfect cure. This is a very important assertion when we remember the thousands of uncured cases now taking their weary journey through life, with that most distressing clog, an uncured ulcer of the leg. Occasionally, however, cases will be found where the skin, or the fresh granulations of the ulcer will not bear the bandage, either because it is directly too painful, or because the patient does not succeed in so applying it as to have it render the service required. But even in these instances, a short discontinuance of its use, and a subsequent careful readjustment, together with particular instructions in regard to its application, will generally remove all difficulties.

It may also be mentioned, that the rubber bandage is frequently found of great service, where there are ordinary varicose veins, without any eczema or ulceration; and, as it can be adjusted day by day to suit the condition of the parts, it is much more manageable and satisfactory to the patient than either the laced or elastic stocking. At first patients may complain of the heat, irritation, and perspiration, but after a few days these will cease to give annoyance, and the comfort of the bandage will be appreciated.

In regard to the bandages themselves, they should be made of the best, selected, pure rubber, as thin as possible, and very elastic. They are ordinarily twelve feet long and three inches wide, as I have employed them; they may be made of any dimensions. On one end, a piece of cloth is cemented, an inch or so wide, to give firm attachment to the tapes which are to tie the free extremity. These tapes should, of course, be rolled inside, and the bandage is prepared for application, exactly as any other roller bandage. The envelopment should invariably be commenced at the toes, or just behind the joint of the large toe, and after one or two turns around the foot, it is passed around the ankle, and back beneath the foot once more, and then continued up the leg; generally the heel may be left uncovered. It is not necessary to reverse the turns, as with the ordinary cotton bandage, for, by a little manipulation the rubber may be readily made to yield so as to be smoothly applied without this twisting, which injures it. In order to have the bandage hold firmly, it should generally extend almost to the knee. In case the eruption reaches above the knee a single bandage will sometimes be sufficient, or if not, a second one may be begun where the first ceases, and thus the envelopment may be made even to the groin. In one of my private patients four bandages were thus worn, two on either leg, with the very best effect and with the result of the perfect cure of a very extensive, severe, and previously obstinate eczema rubrum affecting all of both legs; the patient was a large, fat, middle aged gentleman, who spent much time standing at a desk writing. With a little care these bandages may be worn for a considerable length of time; I have known of many of them which had been worn for more than six months; it is to be remembered that grease or glycerine must not be applied to or left on the skin at the same time, for either will soon destroy the elasticity and worth of the bandage. That this is not necessary will be seen from what is next to be mentioned in regard to their application.

The mode of application of the bandage is comparatively simple, but some attention to details is necessary in order to ensure success in its use. The first care to be exercised is that it be not applied too tightly, for it is possible by means of it to force all of the blood out of a limb, and to quite check the circulation, as when employed in Esmarch's bloodless operation. Ordinarily it need be drawn only just tight enough to perceive that there is the slightest possible stretching of the rubber, no more. I always apply the bandage myself the first time, and have the patient watch very carefully, taking pains to give a little instruction as I make the turns, and I find that even the more ignorant patients in public practice can employ them very satisfactorily. After they are first applied by the physician, they are to be left in place, unless too tight and painful, until the patient retires for the night. In varicose ulcers or where there is much tendency to sluggish circulation in the limb I have them taken off only after the patient is entirely undressed and in bed. On being removed the bandage is to be immersed at once in water, and if the odor is very fœtid this may contain thymol (1 : 1000) or a small proportion of carbolic acid. The legs are to be gently wiped off or washed off with lukewarm water, but with as little exposure and friction as possible, and dried carefully. If there is still a discharging eczematous surface it may be covered with cotton batting, and an ordinary roller bandage or other wrapping very lightly applied for the night. When there is a raw, exuding ulcer it may be protected with a bit of lint spread with any mild ointment, as simple cerate, mutton tallow, or vaseline, to prevent it adhering. All greasy substances must be well but gently removed by wiping in the morning before the application of the rubber bandage.

After the leg is dressed for the night the bandage is to be removed from the water, wiped dry, and hung up to air. In the morning the dressing is to be removed gently from the affected limb, and if cotton has been applied, it is to be carefully pulled off from the surface, without doing violence to the diseased part; that is, the outer portions are gently removed, and fibres which may stick to an exuding surface are left still adherent, though as few of them as possible, and the bandage is re-applied directly over them. Any dressing which has been placed upon an ulceration is to be removed carefully, and the surface very gently wiped to free it of grease, but it is not to be washed off; if the cloth is adherent to the ulcer it should be soaked off with a water-dressing or oil. All this should be done before leaving the bed in the morning, and the bandage is to be re-applied while the patient is still in bed, as the foot should not be put to the floor except when the parts are protected and supported by the bandage. If there is much tendency to varicosity of the veins, or swelling of the limb, we may aid the recovery by slightly elevating the foot of the bedstead by a couple of bricks, that the blood pressure of the limb may be lessened during the hours of sleep. If the leg is very hot and painful with the bandage on, much relief and benefit may be obtained by making cold applications on the outside.

A caution may be here given, in regard to the removal of the bandage. Care must be exercised, not to dispense with it too soon, indeed, it should be worn for a longer or shorter period after the eczema or ulcer is apparently well. When there are varicose veins, patients are very willing, and often even express the desire to continue wearing the bandage, on account of the constant sense of relief to the tense, swollen feeling which is experienced. Another caution may be added with regard to the occasional omission of the bandage during treatment. Very much harm may occur from leaving it off even for a single day, from the blood distension which follows; while, if left off in very cold weather, without equivalent protection, serious results may follow from the exposure to the cold; the tissues being softened by the rubber, the sweat glands having been previously very active, chill of the surface very readily takes place, and I have seen quite serious trouble result from it. In cold weather it might be prudent always to advise some extra protection to the limb for a season after discontinuing the use of the rubber bandage.

A very important point to bear in mind in relation to this mode of treatment is connected with what has been previously said in regard to the physiological conditions of the circulation in the legs. It was shown that the valves in the veins play no unimportant part in aiding the circulation, which is forced on by the contraction of the voluntary muscles. When the patient wears a rubber bandage, this element comes into play to the highest degree; the elastic rubber yields with each motion, and contraction follows expansion. As a rule, therefore, the patient wearing a rubber bandage for lesions of the lower extremity, will be benefited far more than injured by any moderate amount of exercise; I therefore urge my patients thus treated to walk as far as reasonably possible, short of fatigue. This must be advised with caution at first, but after the limb has become accustomed to and benefited by the treatment, patients will experience far more relief and comfort when walking about, than when sitting still. In one instance, a man who had been in an hospital for six weeks, with ulcers and eczema of the leg, with very little improvement to his condition, walked

six miles on the day after the application of this bandage. Another patient, with varicose ulcer of the leg
which was so painful as to confine him to bed, so that the
bandage was applied while there, walked several miles the
day following its application, and remained on his feet
working until cured.

It is hardly possible here, to give contra-indications to
the use of the rubber bandage, so constantly is it found
of service. I have, however, had a few cases where it did
not appear to be of value, or where the patients insisted
that it was not beneficial; but these were rare exceptions,
and I cannot tell the reasons governing them, they appeared quite like the very many others in whom this method was used with advantage. In one instance the patient
was directed to leave some cotton upon an ulcer, and from
ignorance and carelessness she left a considerable mass on
for some length of time, and remained absent from the
clinic. The cotton became saturated with pus, proved
intensely irritating, and from her tight drawing of the
bandage over it she caused a superficial slough, which
gave considerable annoyance and delayed the progress of
the case; but she afterwards wore the bandage with
benefit.

Other measures are more or less of value in conjunction with the treatment of eczema of the leg by means of
the rubber bandage, although in a large share of the cases
the plan which has been detailed affords the best prospects of a speedy and perfect cure, in connection, of
course, with appropriate general measures. Sometimes
the cotton is not an agreeable application after the
removal of the bandage at night; we may then, even
when raw and exuding, dress the diseased part at night
with a mild zinc ointment spread on lint, and laid on. As
in raw eczema elsewhere, the ointment should never be
rubbed upon the affected part. If there is much itching

a small portion of tar may be added to the ointment (Formula 57). But this method of treatment at night has its disadvantages in the tendency of the cloth to adhere to the part, and thus to do violence to the raw surface when removed in the morning; also the ointment or grease which is left upon the limb, will be required to be removed in the morning before the application of the bandage, and this very removal may do harm. This cleansing is best accomplished by firmly but gently wiping the surface with a soft, dry cloth; washing does injury to the newly formed epidermal layer.

Later in the case, when the surface has become dry, and when the circulation is sluggish, and there is still some thickening, we may obtain benefit from the use of the compound tincture of green soap (Formula 41), quickly rubbed on at night, followed by diachylon or other soothing ointment. Rarely is it necessary to use other local measures than these; if carefully applied, they will certainly cure in a comparatively brief period of time, very many of the cases of eczema of the lower leg, if used in conjunction with proper general management.

Where the rubber bandage cannot be procured, or for some reason is not employed, good results can still be obtained by other measures. In cases which are at all severe, rest in a recumbent posture is necessary, indeed in some instances the condition is well nigh incurable unless this can be secured. But when acute symptoms have subsided it is better for the patient to walk if the part is properly supported by a bandage. To obtain the greatest benefit from rest the limb should not only be elevated from the ground, but, even when reclining, the foot should be elevated above the level of the rest of the body; during the day the patient may sit in a low rocking chair, and, leaning back, may have the limb on a table, actually elevated above the level of the heart.

In an acute eruption a lotion is generally most service-able, and the lead and opium, or the calamine wash (Formulæ 31, 32, 39), may be frequently applied; at night an ointment is more appropriate, thickly spread on lint (Formulæ 51, 52, 56), the tarry ointment (Formula 57), is to be used if there is much itching. As the acute character and exudation cease (if the rubber bandage is not employed) a roller bandage of light flannel, or gauze, or cotton should be applied over a suitable ointment spread upon lint, and this dressing made before the patient leaves the bed in the morning. These legs should not be washed much in the ordinary manner, indeed hardly at all except under the conditions and in the manner shortly to be described. In certain cases of sub-acute eczema of the lower extremities, the red, raw, exuding surface does not yield to mildly astringent remedies, such as just indicated, and the best results may be obtained from strapping the entire limb with strips of litharge plaster, as ordinarily done for ulcer of the leg, only to a very much greater extent. If well applied and comfortable, this dressing may remain undisturbed for a day or more; when it becomes loosened and is removed, the surface beneath is found less red and moist, and in cases where this application is found to suit, the progress toward cure is often very rapid.

When the condition has become still more chronic, and there is a thickened, red, and scaly surface, stimulation is necessary, but it must be conducted with caution and in just the right manner or harm will result. The safest stimulants are the compound tincture of green soap and the liquor picis alkalinus (Formulæ 40, 41). These may generally be used in full strength, but should be diluted one or more times with water at the time of first using and upon very delicate skins. They are to be firmly and quickly rubbed over the part with a bit of muslin until some little burning or even pain results; this will be the more readily borne and is even welcomed, as it arrests the itching which is generally very troublesome in these cases. After a thorough rubbing, which will result in the production of excoriated points and consequently in some exudation, the surface is to be gently wiped with a damp cloth, and a soothing ointment applied (Formulæ 51, 52, 61); or, if there is much burning, cold water dressing may be kept on for a while, followed by an ointment.

Greater stimulation can be obtained by stronger solutions of the green soap, sapo viridis, in alcohol or water (Formula 42), or by the use of the soap itself in the manner directed in the chapter upon general treatment, and elsewhere; or, caustic potash may be employed in solution, from five to thirty or more grains to the ounce, applied in the same manner. But care must always be exercised that the stimulation caused by the frictions is allowed to subside perfectly under the proper ointment before it is repeated.

In still more chronic states more stimulant ointments may be used with benefit, and those containing mercury will be found most serviceable (Formulæ 62, 65, 68). The glycerole of the sub-acetate of the lead as brought forward by Mr. Balmanno Squire (Formula 36), is also valuable for these legs presenting a thickening, and a reddened, scaly surface. It is to be used diluted four to ten times with glycerine, or with water and glycerine if the former is too drying.

The local treatment of ulcers of the leg will be found very difficult in a majority of the cases without the rubber bandage: indeed with our present knowledge this means is the one which should invariably be used, unless experience in the individual cases shows it inapplicable.

Where the rubber bandage is not used it will be necessary to keep the limb elevated for a time, but if possible it is better not to heal ulcers by confining the patient in bed, otherwise they are very apt to recur when the upright posture is resumed. The limb should be supported by a well fitting bandage of some kind. Black wash (Formula 34), is often of great service, and gives a considerable measure of relief in ulcers of the leg. The sore is to be frequently wet with it; and a piece of cloth saturated with the same is kept on the part during the day time; at night a slightly stimulating ointment (Formula 69), is laid on, spread upon lint, and the foot of the bed slightly elevated on bricks. In removing a dressing from an ulcer it is desirable to avoid irritating the surface by tearing it off, if adherent; it is best therefore to use the ointment very freely in a thick layer, in order to prevent the cloth from sticking to the ulcerated surface.

Many plans of treatment of ulcer of the leg have been advocated from time to time and are suitable in selected cases; it would be impossible even to mention them all in this connection. All are intended to fulfil the same end, namely support to distended and weakened vessels, protection to exposed and irritated surfaces, relief from the pain, and, gentle and proper stimulation to indolent tissues. The common method of strapping with diachylon plaster is of value; to be efficient the straps should extend around the limb so as to lap over and give support.

Lotions of chloral half a drachm to a drachm in the pint of water, squeezed over the ulcer night and morning, will relieve much of the pain: the ulcer is then to be lightly dressed with a soothing ointment. Chlorate of potash in about the same strength also improves the condition of the ulcer and promotes healing.

Some caution must be exercised in using the nitrate of silver as a caustic to ulcers of the leg; if this is rubbed freely over the surface, as is sometimes done, the fresh epidermic formations from the sides will be destroyed and the process of healing will be proportionately delayed. The ulcer should, therefore, be carefully touched, and the cauterization should not go further than to within a slight distance of its edges. Indolent ulcers may sometimes be stimulated into healthy action and to healing by the application of a fly blister, and although it is extremely difficult to obtain anything like its characteristic action on the surface, it is often followed by great benefit.

Epidermic grafting must never be forgotten in the treatment of obstinate eczematous or varicose ulceration ; if properly carried out it serves a good end in affording points of cicatrization when the granulations are not disposed to form epidermic tissue.

The internal treatment of ulcers by opium, given especially at night in doses quite sufficient to subdue the pain, is one which often proves most valuable. Care should always be exercised to avoid constipation from this, otherwise much harm may result.

Eczema about the ankles and on the upper part of the foot generally requires pretty severely stimulating measures, and may prove rebellious even to these. Beginning with the compound tincture of green soap, we may increase the strength of the application, using the liquor picis alkalinus (Formula 40), pure or diluted a few times. Or, caustic potassa solutions five to twenty or more grains to the ounce ; or tincture of iodine, and perhaps solutions of nitrate of silver. Some care must be exercised not to carry the matter of stimulation too far, but generally eczema of these parts will be found to resist pretty severe measures.

On the under surface of the toes and sides of the feet we sometimes have a sub-acute eczema, characterized by the repeated development of vesicles, accompanied with a considerable degree of itching and often with a soreness which renders walking painful. This generally ceases upon the continued application of the diachylon ointment, spread thickly on lint, or yields to a tarry ointment (Formula 57), aided by foot baths containing tannin. I also have seen most excellent results from opening the vesicles as fast as they are formed, and keeping the surface well dusted with the acetate of aluminium. Eczema between the toes may be very distressing and rebellious, owing to the confined secretion of the parts, the pressure of the foot coverings, and the constant movements of the joints. The principles to be followed in its management are to keep the affected toes separated by strips of muslin spread with ointment, generally the diachylon, and, while preserving cleanliness, to avoid irritation by washing; it is generally best to cleanse the parts by gentle wiping. Foot baths of white oak bark infusion, or tannin are serviceable. I have seen very excellent results from dusting the parts with the acetate of aluminium.

Dry eczema of the soles of the feet presents much the same appearances, and the diagnostic features are the same as in eczema of the palms, and for this reference can be made to the preceding chapter. The treatment is also much the same. An additional method, often of great service in these cases, is the constant wearing of oiled-silk, which may be cut of the proper size and sewed within the stocking; this is worn night and day, the stocking being changed at night, turned inside out, and left to dry and air. The constant maceration of the parts tends to remove the thickening, and gives great relief to the patient.

Eczema of other portions of the limb is to be treated in the manner described for eczema of a similar character upon other locations of the body. Where the eruption is at all extensive, alkaline baths (Formula 27), followed by a carbolic acid ointment (Formula 73), are of the greatest service. A tarry oil (Formula 49), often answers very well as a local application, thoroughly but gently rubbed into the part. Proper occasional stimulation is often called for, with subsequent protection, as with tar and zinc ointment (Formula 57), to which a little citrine ointment may be added, if the patches are hard and resisting. Chronic papular eczema of the thighs and legs, where the papules are either discrete and generally scattered, or gathered into patches or circles, will sometimes prove very rebellious and require very severe stimulation, although generally alkaline baths repeated daily, with the subsequent use of the oil alluded to will suffice, with internal measures, to remove the eruption. The itching of even a moderate eczema on the legs, is sometimes exceedingly severe, and no little trouble will be experienced in allaying it. In such cases chloral and camphor combined with a powder or ointment (Formulæ 25, 71), are of service ; also liquor potassæ and glycerine (Formula 43).

Eczema on the upper and inner portions of the thighs and its management, will be treated of in the next chapter in connection with eczema of the anus and genital region.

CHAPTER XIII.

THE MANAGEMENT OF ECZEMA OF THE ANUS AND GENITAL REGION.

THE misery endured by patients affected at all severely with eczema about the anus and genital region, can be but little understood except by those who have thus suffered, or who have had much to do with those affected with the same. Cases of the eruption in this locality are far more common than may be imagined, or than appears from statistics, and the many instances constantly met with where the eruption has already lasted a great length of time, indicate that the importance of the disease in this locality, is not fully appreciated by the profession, and that the measures which will give permanent relief are not as well understood as they might be.

Of the twelve hundred cases of eczema occurring in private practice, there were one hundred and fifty-four in which these parts were invaded, or more than twelve per cent. of the entire number. The records of the dispensary and hospital cases have not been kept with sufficient minuteness to allow of analyzing them in this respect, but from the very many instances which constantly occur in public practice, I think I do not exaggerate in placing the ratio of the cases of eczema in this region to those where other portions of the body are affected at not less than one-tenth of all cases of this disease. But even this figure probably does not represent by any means the real frequency of the eruption in this location, for sufferers from eczema of the anus or genital region often if not generally hide their trouble until it has lasted long and has become unendurable; this is especially true in regard to females, as is also shown by the fact that a very large share of the cases which have come under my care have been in males. The reasons for this concealment are numerous and easily understood. Shame undoubtedly prevents many from exposing diseases of these parts to the knowledge of others; the idea is more or less prevalent, that any disease in this region may have some connection with sexual transgressions. Again many with eczema of the anus, imagine that they have piles; indeed, many cases of this trouble very often pass among the general profession as " itching piles," while, of course, every disease about the anus is thus named by the " pile doctors," to whom these unfortunates often apply. Eczema about the genital folds also often passes for simple chafing, until it is deep seated and the long continuance of the causes and results have induced a condition very difficult to cure. Many cases also go untreated because of the impression that but little can be done for affections of the skin.

Eczema of the anus and genital region, does not differ essentially from the same disease as manifested elsewhere, but there are certain peculiar features about it which demand especial consideration, and there are certain elements in its management which require very particular description; for it is in the details of practice that the difference lies between success and want of success.

Acute eczema of the anus is not very common, except when it occurs by extension from other parts, when we may have it acutely developed here as well as elsewhere. As a rule, however, it is insidiously developed, and very rarely do we find any of the phenomena belonging to the state described elsewhere as acute inflammatory eczema. About the genitals, however, we may and frequently do have a more or less acutely developed eruption, either alone or in connection with eczema of other parts. The genitals will then be the seat of greater or less redness, heat, and œdematous swelling, with perhaps the formation of papules or vesicles ; more commonly, however, we meet with only the erythematous eczema.

All degrees and grades of chronic eczema may be observed in the regions under consideration ; and sometimes those cases which present the least external evidence of the disease may give rise to the most suffering.

About the anus the lesion sometimes consists in but a slight amount of thickening of the muco-cutaneous surface, with a little purplish congestion, and perhaps rather a few superficial excoriations on or between the folds of the part; and yet the distress with itching and pain may be intense and may be the cause of greatly disturbed sleep, or it may even rob the patient of peace and comfort. But the really severe cases show, of course, manifold more external signs of the disease, and the entire anal and genital region may be the seat of a greatly thickened, moist, exuding surface extending on either side of the nates, for an inch or more. Very often the condition seen is a whitened, soggy state of the parts between the buttocks, with or without some excoriated points, and with a thickening and deepening of the natural furrows in the mucous membrane about the anus. This condition gives rise not only to periodical or permanent itching, but may even cause great pain on sitting, or during defecation.

This state may affect the region of the anus alone, or may extend to and involve the entire male or female genital region as well ; or, these latter may be affected alone even to a very severe degree, without the process extending to the region of the anus. Eczema in this location is by no means always associated with the same on other parts of the body; in some of the worst cases which I have been called upon to treat, there has been no sign of cutaneous disease except upon the anus or genitals, or both. Although I have also frequently seen it associated with a similar eruption elsewhere, or with the history of preceding eczema of other parts.

Chronic eczema of the scrotum may be general or local. Often the anterior portion alone is involved, or the eruption may attack the under surface of the penis and extend along the raphe, even to the anus. When affected most severely there may be very considerable swelling, which consists of infiltration or thickening of tissue, with some œdema; if pinched between the fingers the skin is found to be thickened, even to many times its normal state. The eruption in this locality is usually of the erythematous variety, with no vesicles and even with no moisture, but with only redness and thickening, accompanied by intense itching. On the sides of the scrotum where it lies against the thighs the skin is more apt to take on the moist form, and may become quite raw.

There is also another condition not infrequent on the sides of the scrotum in eczema cases, in which there appear white, solid papules, of some size, often discharging a little pus, and quite sore; these appear to be closed and inflamed follicles, and are of little significance, as they disappear under the proper treatment for the disease. Fissures are seldom seen upon the scrotum.

Eczema of the penis is generally seen in the erythematous form; the prepuce alone may be affected, or the disease may involve the entire organ and extend well on to the pubis. The glans may also be affected, presenting a hard, scaly, and itchy surface. There is always more or less of œdema associated with eczema of the penis, and sometimes this may be very considerable, and be the cause of some little anxiety. The itching also of eczema of this part is exceedingly distressing, and generally causes the patient to rub and pinch the part many times a day.

Eczema may sometimes extend from the anus and genitals well into the crotch, and sometimes even down on the thighs, but this is unusual; very commonly when the eruption spreads thus upon the thighs and crotch, it will be found to be what is called eczema marginatum, a ringworm of this region, which will be more particularly described shortly when we come to speak of diagnosis. We not infrequently however, do have true eczema developing first in the crotch alone and reaching thence to a greater or less extent upon the thigh, also sometimes upon the scrotum on one or both sides; this often begins as a simple chafing or intertrigo, and in proper subjects develops in intensity, until it becomes an affair of importance and gives much distress. Intertrigo or eczema of this region also often affords the nidus upon which may develop later the parasitic eczema marginatum, as will be described hereafter.

Eczema of the female genitals, may likewise exist alone or in connection with eczema of other parts, or may come by extension of the eruption from the anal region. Here we may observe it in the most varied degrees, from a slight vesiculo-papular lesion upon the labia, giving but little annoyance and only occasionally itching a little, even up to one which may involve the entire region of the pubis and upper thighs, causing an amount of misery impossible to describe and scarcely to be believed except by those who have experienced it. In milder cases the true condition may readily escape recognition, and the trouble may pass for pruritus. But careful examination will show the external or internal labia to be harsh and dry, and the seat of inflammatory reddening and thickening, and probably they will exhibit a greater or less number of excoriated points. The eruption may also extend for some distance

up the vagina. In more severe cases the labia often become the seat of enormous hypertrophic thickening, the
surface being hard and papular, and also the seat of many
abrasions, from the continued scratching and rubbing of
the part. Eczema marginatum must also be looked for
in the female as well as in the male, and may exist as a
complication of what had previously been ordinary eczema.
Eczema about the female genitals frequently arises as a
secondary eruption, consequent upon the scratching which
may have preceded from itching due to irritating vaginal
or uterine secretions, or in connection with glycosuria.

Many of the cases of eczema in the regions under
consideration frequently pass as pruritus or even prurigo
of these parts, but in by far the larger share of the cases
ordinarily regarded as such, the cause of the itching will
be found to be really an eczema, which sooner or later will
or does develop into more characteristic features.

The diagnosis of eczema of the anus and genital
region should not ordinarily present very great difficulty,
if care be taken. But there are several conditions which
it is well always to bear in mind in order to a perfect understanding and successful treatment of these cases.

It is desirable always as a matter of routine to eliminate the possibility of the eruption being due to pediculi,
for these may sometimes be found even in the highest
walks of life, and may give rise to an itching which closely
resembles that of eczema, and the subsequent scratching
may cause abrasions simulating this eruption. It is quite
possible, of course, that crab-lice might be present only as
a complication, but it is well to ascertain the fact, for if
present they could act as a local cause which would prolong the trouble greatly. A little care will always discover
the nits upon the hairs, if they exist, and generally the insects may be found adhering to the hairs, close to the
skin, and seeming almost like small scabs, so firmly do
they cling by their crab-like claws.

Scabies should also always be borne in mind, for in males some lesions are very commonly found on the penis and scrotum, and occasionally in scabies the region of the lower abdomen will be the seat of very considerable papular eruption, and the itching and scratching may extend to the parts beneath. Generally, however, the signs of scabies are abundant elsewhere, and when they do occur on the penis or scrotum, the lesions are seen to be single, isolated, rather shotty papules, and often the cuniculus or furrow of the insect can be discovered in connection with them. It must also be remembered that in cases of scabies which have been submitted to severe treatment, the genital region may become considerably irritated by the treatment itself, and an artificial inflammation may be left, resembling eczema.

The most important eruption to remember in connection with eczema of the anus and genital region is that which has already been alluded to as eczema marginatum, which is in reality not an eczema, but a vegetable parasitic eruption, or ring-worm of these parts, known as tinea trichophytina cruris. This may often occur independently, or it may exist as a complication of a pre-existing eczema, and not infrequently we observe at one and the same time the characteristics of the parasitic disease, combined with those of eczema.

This so-called eczema marginatum has a feature belonging to ring-worm, of which it is but one of the forms, which, if sufficient attention is given to it, can generally be made out with sufficient accuracy to make the diagnosis comparatively simple and certain. This is its tendency to advance peripherally with a sharply defined margin, while the surface behind clears up more or less, leaving a brownish, slightly scaly surface. Eczema does not present this sharply defined margin, nor has it the tendency to disappear in parts over which it has passed;

so that in the case of eczema in the crotch we find the most severely marked disease at the fork of the thigh, and the eruption rather fades towards its outer portion, exactly the reverse of that which is found in eczema marginatum. Sometimes, or perhaps generally, in eczema marginatum in males, we find a patch or patches upon one or both sides of the scrotum, exactly coinciding in shape and dimensions with those upon the thigh. And in females sometimes the two thighs for a little distance are attacked symmetrically. Or in the case of the abdomen in fat persons with pendulous bellies, there may be a ring upon opposite surfaces where two surfaces of skin come in contact.

This eczema marginatum may also extend upon the anal region, and we have then on either side of the buttocks where they touch each other, a sharply defined, red, marginal line, with comparatively little redness or with a soggy condition of the parts within it. As previously mentioned, this parasitic eruption may occur as a complication of eczema of this region, and what was previously an ordinary eczema without any sharply defined margin, may by the advent of the parasite, take on the form here described. But in certain cases, on the other hand, the parasitic eruption may be of old date, and the eczema may develop upon it from the severity of the itching and the consequent scratching, or from the stimulant applications given to relieve it. On several occasions in females I have seen an eczema arise from the pruritus attendant upon glycosuria, and a parasitic eczema marginatum then develop upon the simple eczema. Unless this parasitic eruption is recognized and met therapeutically, the case will prove most rebellious. The existence of a tolerably well defined margin, or perhaps of simply outlying, circular patches, or the occurrence of newly developed patches of various sizes within an area previously affected on this region of the body near the crotch, should always lead to the suspicion of the existence of this parasitic disease. The surface should then be gently scraped with a rather dull knife, and the scales and debris placed in a little liquor potassæ and glycerine, under a magnifying power of three hundred diameters. It is not, however, always as easy to discover the parasite as would be thought; but a little care and time, and familiarity with the subject, will generally reveal the presence of the spores and mycelium of a vegetable parasite among and in the scales, if present. If not found in the first specimen examined, the operation should be repeated.

On a number of occasions, I have seen syphilitic lesions about the anus and genital regions, both mucous patches and papular and tubercular eruptions, which have been called eczema and treated as such ; and this not only in the case of infantile syphilis, but also in adults. The lesions of the two are so entirely different, when carefully considered, that they should never be confounded.

Herpes of the genital organs is more frequently mistaken for venereal ulcers, but it may likewise resemble eczema in a measure, and the two should be differentiated. Here we have little groups of vesicles upon a slightly inflamed base, with some burning, but not much if any itching; these reappear easily, and if not irritated pass away spontaneously in a few days.

Finally, many cases of pruritus of these parts, undoubtedly do occur, which should not be classed as eczema, although, as remarked before, some cases are probably classed as pruritus and prurigo of these regions which are in reality eczema. In pruritus of the scrotum, there will be the entire absence of thickening and redness, and only the marks of scratching will be seen ; and generally these are not abundant, because relief is very generally obtained more readily than in eczema, by simply pinching the part, and severe scratching and tearing the surface is not indulged in as when eczema is present. Pruritus of the anus may sometimes give rise to so much distress that the parts are torn severely, and the suffering from pruritus of the vulva and vagina may occasionally be beyond description. But many of these cases, where at first sight there appears to be only itching, are in reality in the very earliest stage of eczema, or are slightly pronounced cases of the same, and, unless this fact is recognized they frequently go unrelieved. When, however, the itching is due to an early or slightly developed eczema, very much more can be done than in many cases of true pruritus; indeed the trouble can be removed entirely.

The prognosis of eczema of the anus and genital region must vary somewhat with the case ; but the condition is, in the main, curable. The more severe cases are often much more manageable than those presenting less actual features of the disease, and the most aggravated cases, which have lasted for months, or perhaps for years, may, with exactly the right treatment, yield in as many days or weeks.

The etiology of eczema in the locations under consideration is, in general, the same as that affecting other portions of the body: it is not a purely local disease, but has the constitutional relations which have been previously detailed with regard to eczema elsewhere. Indeed the local causes are more difficult to discover and demonstrate here than in regard to eczema of almost any other region of the body; the eruption will come most unexpectedly, and no adequate local cause can generally be made out, although there are some elements which probably are of etiological importance in certain cases. In regard to eczema of the anus, it is quite possible that an irritating condition of the secretions of the parts may be the exciting cause in some instances ; also, possibly an acrid state of the intestinal discharges may excite the eruption. The passage of greatly

hardened fæces may also irritate the parts. The use of
improper and irritating water-closet paper, also very rough
underclothing, may act as local excitants. Eczema of the
scrotum can arise from irritation or chafing from underclothing, or horseback riding, or possibly from an irritating
character of the secretions of the part. Eczema of the
penis sometimes follows upon a gonorrhœal discharge.

Eczema of the female genitals, perhaps not infrequently,
has its local cause in the irritating nature of the vaginal or
urinal secretions. Eczema of this region may be owing to
the irritation of intestinal worms, though this appears to be
a very infrequent cause.

But all these, perhaps many more, local causes may exist
in certain individuals and yet never provoke an eczema,
and they may even have occurred to the same person on
previous occasions, and yet not have caused the eruption.
There is certainly some other state or element which requires to be recognized and met in order to give these
patients perfect and permanent relief.

The most common general symptom observed in patients with eczema of the anal or genital region, is constipation, or, as it might be more properly called, imperfect
intestinal excretion, generally with faulty liver action. This
indeed almost invariably exists to a greater or less extent
in these cases, and requires to be looked for and managed
properly. So commonly have I found this in the very considerable number of cases of eczema of the anus and genital region which have come under my care, that I would
almost declare it to be an invariable accompaniment of this
condition; but on going over my notes of cases, I find a
certain small proportion of instances in which it is stated
by the patient that the bowels act regularly once or twice
daily. This, however, is not convincing proof that the
intestinal action is perfect, and I still believe this element
to be the most important single factor in the disease; for

there may undoubtedly be one or more movements of the bowels in the day, and yet the intestinal secretion may not represent that of health. Not at all infrequently do I find, on closer questioning, that the character of the secretions is unhealthy, too dark or too light colored, often accompanied with wind ; or that they are fœtid, etc.

This imperfect intestinal excretion should be corrected if possible, and very great care will sometimes be necessary to accomplish this, as was mentioned in the chapter on general treatment. It is not enough to give occasional purgatives, nor even to prescribe daily laxatives, for, unless much caution is exercised, the ultimate result in this direction may be bad instead of good. This, and the remarks on this subject in this and other chapters in regard to the management of this important element in the disease under consideration, may seem trite and out of place, but I wish to impress the very great importance of dealing with this portion of the management rightly, as a *sine qua non* of the successful management of eczema in the parts under consideration. All the elements which conduce to bring about a healthy action of the bowels and organs of digestion must therefore be attended to, and consequently in the treatment of eczema about the anus and genitals, we must not be content with a few general questions and directions, or with the prescription of one or another purgative or laxative remedy. On the contrary it may require no little trouble to insure a healthy evacuation of the bowels every day, and yet this must be accomplished. To this end attention is to be directed to diet, exercise, regularity in attending to the calls of nature, etc., while such assistance as may be necessary is to be given by means of medicines.

A very common accompaniment of eczema of the anus and genital region is a greater or less congestion of the portal and hemorrhoidal circulation, manifested by a purplish congestion of the mucous membrane of the anus, or, very commonly, by a greater or less degree of internal or external piles. These latter may not be sufficient to be recognized by the patient, and yet be an element indicative of an existing state of the internal organs which must be met and rectified. It is well, therefore, in examining patients thus affected, to have them strain or bear down, in order to bring the deeper portions to view. When this congestion of the hemorrhoidal vessels exists, I almost invariably give the time-honored mixture of precipitated sulphur and cream of tartar (Formula 20) in quantities sufficient to secure one or two loose movements from the bowels daily. I never give it with syrup, as I believe this often ferments, or acts prejudicially on the stomach, and in a measure impairs the good effects desired. One or two teaspoonfuls of the mixture are to be taken each night on retiring, rubbed up with a little water into a paste. The dose is not a very pleasant one, but it is readily taken even by ladies. This should be continued for some length of time, perhaps even for weeks, the dose being varied somewhat according to the results produced; but the amount taken daily should be as uniform as possible, it being gradually diminished as the desired effect is produced, which is never to be a severe purgation, but only the securing of one or two rather loose stools. So commonly useful is this in eczema about the anus and genitals, that I frequently order it even when a decided hemorrhoidal congestion is not observed. It is hardly supposed that the sulphur acts in any special way upon the eczema, except through its action on the liver and intestinal secretions.

As a laxative in the beginning of the treatment of eczema in this region, the pill of blue mass, colocynth, and ipecac (Formula 13) gives excellent results; two such pills are taken at night, one at nine and one at ten o'clock, and two on the second night after, followed each morning by a Seidlitz powder, or Kissingen water. This saline, however, is not necessary, and I frequently omit it. These pills should be taken only twice, and are not to be resorted to continually, although they may be used at an interval of a week or so with good effect, if necessary.

If there is simply a sluggish action of the bowels, I have often had most excellent results to the accompanying eczema from the use of a pill composed of aloes and iron (Formula 14), one pill being taken directly after eating; or, when other medicine is given after eating, the pill may be taken before the meal. Very much may be accomplished by this combination in the way of permanently overcoming the constipated habit, if the pills are employed regularly and systematically according to the following directions: At first one pill or more is taken three times daily; in a few days the noon dose is omitted or diminished, and a few days later, as regular action of the bowels is established, the number employed is further diminished, so that but one pill is taken at the time of the evening meal only, and soon this is required less frequently, and subsequently discontinued. The point to be insisted on is that the pills shall be used regularly in the above manner until the bowels acquire the habit of daily excreting and discharging a normal amount; if they are taken irregularly, simply for a cathartic action, no ultimate good results will follow. But I can bear testimony very strongly to the value of this plan of treatment, which I have followed for years, and could attest from many cases that this has constituted one of the chief means of speedy and permanent cure of long standing eczema of the anus and genital region.

It is a very common custom with many, to give medicinal waters to these patients, with the simple direction that they keep the bowels open therewith. In my experience this is an unwise procedure, as mentioned in a previous chapter, and I believe that many persons are to-day suffering from constipation, and consequent eczema of the lower

region of the body, because of the constant stimulation of
the intestinal tract with these or other purgatives, while the
cause of the intestinal inactivity, such as sedentary habits,
over-indulgence at the table, etc., have been allowed to go
on unchecked.   Nor is it sufficient in these cases simply
to secure an emptying of the lower bowel by means of an
enema, as has also been previously alluded to; if employed at
all, in my judgment, enemata are to be used only very rarely,
for definite purposes, and the habit of dependence on water
injected into the bowels to excite the intestines to contraction, is worse even than having them depend on mineral
waters poured into the other end of the digestive tube.
Nor will an action of the bowels secured by an enema, at
all help an eczema of the anal or genital region: I have
seen some very bad cases of the eruption in this locality
where this was practiced with great regularity.   The mixture of magnesia and iron (Formula 1), often renders very
great service in these cases; if when taken three times
daily after the meals there is still insufficient action of the
bowels, an additional dose may be given before breakfast,
largely diluted.   If this can be taken with hot water, its
action upon the bowels is all the more full and satisfactory.

Other measures may, undoubtedly, be of much service
in meeting this feature of constipation in these cases, but I
have preferred, in this as in other matters, to mention the
methods which have yielded me the best results, without
attempting to exhaust the subject by reference to others.
Attention to details in this, as in very many of the points
connected with the treatment of diseases of the skin, is of
the greatest importance, and he will but poorly treat these
cases who contents himself with prescribing, in a routine
manner, this or that remedy which has been proposed or
vaunted by however high an authority.   He will also but
poorly manage the intestinal excretion who is satisfied with
giving an occasional casual prescription to loosen the

bowels; the utmost ignorance as to the laws of health is constantly observed in patients, and the physician must give definite instructions on all points in order to insure success.

Next to imperfect bowel excretion has been placed deficient kidney action, as an element to be regarded in the management of eczema, and this is especially true in regard to the cases under consideration. The urine of these patients is seldom that of health ; most varied conditions may be reported, although not at all infrequently the alteration from health is only discovered by chemical or microscopical examination. Often the patient will report the urine as being scanty and high colored, depositing in and staining the chamber; or, he will complain of frequent and imperative micturition, and the repeated calls to urinate at night, together with the itching will often act and react on each other, rendering sleep almost impossible.

These cases, therefore, will receive the greatest benefit from an alkali, and the one I commonly use is the acetate of potassa (Formulæ 2, 3, 6). This is often given at the beginning, and continued during the entire course of treatment, and frequently for some time after the complete disappearance of the eruption and cessation of all itching. Other alkalies may also be used with advantage, as the citrate of potassa (Formula 4) or liquor potassæ alone or with a little belladonna.

Not infrequently, however, cases of eczema of the anus and genitals may be associated with a large amount of oxaluria; and these patients will be quickest relieved by the use of strong nitric acid internally, or muriatic acid, in doses of from two to five minims after meals. In some cases the disease appears to be largely due to simple debility : and iron and other tonics which give life and tone to the system, will do the most good to the eczema. These often act by means of rendering the process of assimilation and disassimilation more perfect, whereby the liver, bowels and kidneys share the healthful activity ; but in these cases careful attention must assuredly be given to the intestinal excretions, otherwise all remedies are useless.

It will be noticed, perhaps, that arsenic has not been mentioned. Yet I am positive that many general practitioners would give arsenic at the first visit to one suffering from the conditions under consideration. I will say, that I did not purposely omit mentioning arsenic, but that it had not occurred to me to speak of it, because, probably, I so seldom prescribe it for these cases. When there is a marked eczematous habit, and when after all of the above measures have been faithfully attended to, and others, perhaps, in the same line, there should still remain a tendency to the disease, arsenic may be employed with advantage, alone or in connection with other remedies. But it can never be used successfully as a curative measure at the beginning of a case, and especially never in cases presenting acute symptoms. As a modifier of the nutrition of the skin, arsenic holds a high place among other medicines, but not as a controller of congestion or of inflammatory action.

If internal and general measures are necessary in eczema of the anus and genital region, proper local treatment is, if possible, of even greater importance. Here, especially, it is much not to do the wrong thing, and still more to do just the right thing. One occasionally sees cases which have been greatly aggravated by previous treatment, which yield promptly to proper measures.

The first main point to be ever borne in mind in the treatment of eczema of these parts, is that more harm than good may often be done by too strong applications, and that the soothing plan must be followed as far as possible, certainly while there are signs of inflammation. Stimulating measures are to be adopted only in later stages of treatment, and to remove the remains of the disease, the thickening of the skin, and not for the arrest of the eczema. Although I have said that acute eczema is not very common in these regions, still all cases present more or less of the features of acute disease, and care must be exercised not to do harm to parts which very readily take on inflammation.

The itching of these cases is often most intense, and the patients will plead that if only something can be given to stop the itching, the disease will get well. And so cases occur in which all sorts and kinds of measures have been prescribed, with a view of arresting the itching, but in vain, whereas these same cases frequently yield speedily when complete and perfect treatment is instituted, including only comparatively mild local measures. Quite recently a physician brought a patient in consultation, not in regard to any general management of the case but only to have my opinion in regard to the probable utility of applying the actual or galvanic cautery to the parts with a view of arresting the itching. And so I have had cases which had been previously given stronger and stronger local applications with a view of checking the itching, until the parts had been brought to a terrible state of inflammation, from such applications .as strong citrine and sulphur ointment, and the like.

The measure which I place most reliance upon, as a means of relieving the congestion of the parts, and the consequent itching, is hot water. But the water should be indeed hot, and not warm ; so hot that the hand cannot be thrust wholly into it, and it should be used exactly in the manner now to be described. The patient should sit on the edge of a chair with a basin of very hot water, and a soft handkerchief in it, on the floor beneath. The handkerchief is picked up and held in a mass to the anus or genital parts, as hot as can be borne, say for a minute, and then dipped into the water again, and the process repeated

about three times. The whole operation should last but a
few minutes, certainly not more than five—perhaps two or
three minutes are generally sufficient. Tepid water, too
long bathing, or too frequent sopping of the part, or rubbing with a cloth, etc., may aggravate the trouble.

Before the hot water is gotten ready, the ointment which
is to be applied should be spread thickly on the woolly
side of surgeon's lint, cut of a size to cover the affected
parts only, and laid close by ready for immediate use.
After the parts have been soaked with the hot water for
the prescribed time, they are rapidly dried by pressing a
large, soft, linen napkin on them, absolutely no friction
being used. The cloths spread with ointment are immediately applied, the object being at once to exclude the
air entirely.

Ordinarily it is necessary to use the hot water only a
single time in the twenty-four hours, namely after undressing and when quite ready to get into bed. It must be
premised that the patient is so to manage as not to indulge
in the usual scratching before undergoing these manipulations; if this desire is given way to beforehand, the treatment will not always control the itching at once. If the
patient can avoid even touching the parts except as described, he or she will commonly be quite able to go to
sleep, immediately after the application. I have repeatedly
had those thus afflicted, say that the first night of treatment
was the first real rest they had had for months or years.

If the case is very severe, that is, if there is very
much thickening or infiltration, and if there is great
itching, the hot water may be repeated occasionally; but it
is commonly sufficient simply to renew the ointment once
or more times in the day, especially in the morning on
arising, without the repetition of the hot water. If used
too frequently, or if the parts are soaked for too long a
time, the hot water sometimes acts prejudicially, by soften-

ing and weakening the parts, as I have repeatedly observed in individuals who, in mistaken zeal, have made the application for a very much longer time than had been directed. It should be added, that the ointment must invariably be spread upon lint, and never be rubbed to the part; also, that in applying the lint it should be kept in close apposition to the diseased surface, and that by means calculated to heat the parts as little as possible. And, finally, it is important that in rearranging the dressing a fresh cloth should be spread and made ready near by before the previous one is removed, that the access of air to the parts may be prevented by changing the coverings as quickly as possible. These parts should not be washed, even for cleanliness, other than as above described. It is often well to have the patient leave on the dressing which has been worn all night, until after stool in the morning; the parts are then carefully wiped with good paper, and other cloths, freshly spread with ointment, are to be instantly reapplied.

The ointment employed must vary somewhat with the case, and no single one could be mentioned which would invariably be of service. That which I most commonly prescribe first, however, is the one so frequently mentioned in connection with eczema of other parts, namely, that containing tar and zinc (Formula 57). If the tar ointment is well made, this should be of a consistency which spreads easily, remains tolerably soft, and adheres fairly well. The solidity of it may be easily regulated by varying the proportion of the spermaceti in the rose ointment or cold cream. I may add that I never employ the recent products of petroleum, cosmoline and vaseline as the basis for these ointments, where protection of the surface and exclusion of the air is desired, as it has not body enough to remain as a thick coating on the lint, but rapidly soaks in, and leaves the diseased surfaces dry and exposed.

While the ointment is not a matter of indifference, equally good results can be obtained by other remedies than the one mentioned. But whatever local treatment is adopted, the method of application is all-important, and strict attention to the details given are necessary for success, which will certainly follow if all the elements alluded to are carried out, including, of course, constitutional hygienic, and other measures. Diachylon, bismuth, zinc, or tannin ointment (Formulæ 52, 53, 54, 61), answer very well, but generally a portion of tar is necessary to assist in allaying the pruritus. Belladonna is often of service in relieving the itching of these parts, and aconite may be added (Formula 72) to heighten the antipruritic effect.

In regard to the employment of stronger local measures in eczema of the anus, it must be premised as of the eruption elsewhere, that the matter of stimulation should be not overdone; although active measures are not infrequently of value in proper cases and at the proper time or period in the disease, if injudiciously used they do harm. When congestion has ceased, and there is still some thickening and a tendency to cutaneous fissures about the anus, we may use the green soap, in simple tincture or combined with the oil of cade (Formulæ 41, 42). To obtain the best results from this it should be applied with some little friction, at first with a bit of muslin and later with white flannel wet with the lotion and rubbed briskly over the parts for a few moments, which are then to be dried and the proper ointment applied; or, if the burning be severe, a damp cloth is laid on for a moment and the part at once covered with a mild ointment. For this purpose the ordinary zinc ointment, half a drachm to the ounce, or the subnitrate of bismuth ointment, or calamine, either in the same strength, may be used; likewise the diachylon ointment, although this appears to be too stimulating for some skins. It is quite as well not to have any tar in these ointments, because having stimulated with a tar lotion the parts want complete rest.

We may sometimes obtain excellent results from caustic potassa in solution, used in much the same way. A lotion of five or ten grains to the ounce is all that can be borne in many instances, but if carefully applied, especially by the physician, one of the strength of fifteen, thirty, or even sixty grains to the ounce may be quickly brushed over the parts; this causes an exudation which is followed by relief of itching, and a diminution of the disease. These strong applications, however, are to be advised with great caution, and care should be taken that soothing measures, as cold-water dressings are afterwards employed, if there is much burning or inflammatory action from the caustic.

When a tendency to slight fissures of the muco-cutaneous folds of the anus still remains, we will have great benefit from touching the latter with a stick of pure nitrate of silver and afterwards packing in a little cotton around the parts. But I must advise this also with caution, because one of the worst cases of acute eczema of the scrotum and anus which I ever had under my care, and which had confined a gentleman to bed for several weeks before I saw him, was started up by having an old eczema of the anus thus touched with caustic, by a gentleman of great eminence in the profession. I have also, myself, seen considerable inflammation excited by a similar application which I had made. If, however, the subsequent inflammation is not too severe, it generally results in great ultimate benefit to the parts. In some cases painting the parts with a solution of nitrate of silver in sweet spirits of nitre, five to twenty grains to the ounce, will be of service, if cautiously used.

The foregoing directions in regard to local applications have referred rather to the management of eczema of the anus; we will now speak more particularly with reference

to that affecting the genital region. Acute eczema of the
penis and scrotum seldom gives much difficulty, and the
avoidance of irritation with the envelopment of the part in
a weak zinc ointment with five or ten drops of carbolic
acid in the ounce, is usually all that is necessary. In the
more chronic state the hot-water plan, previously detailed,
is of the greatest service; the scrotum may be suspended
in a cup of hot water for a few moments, but the plan of
applying the hot water with a soft cloth is generally the
best. The same tar and zinc ointment (Formula 57) is of
the greatest value in eczema of the penis and scrotum, and
is frequently all that will be required. In milder cases, a
lotion may be applied to these parts, with very excellent
effect, and for this purpose one of those containing a
powder, such as that of calamine and zinc (Formulæ 31,32),
to which a little lead water may be added (Formula 35),
answers very well. Hydrocyanic acid (Formula 33) forms
a valuable antipruritic in these cases, but care should be
taken in using it that the surface is not abraded. In the
more chronic state, diluted citrine ointment may be carefully used, alone or with the addition of oil of cade (Formulæ 60, 64, 65). When the thickening and itching persists,
the part may be greatly benefited by the application of a
tarry oil; either the pure oil of cade or the oil of birch
(oleum rusci) may be painted over the part and the hot
water applied over it; or it may be used diluted (Formula 49)
with oil, or as a tincture with equal quantity of alcohol.
This is often, however, a pretty severe application, and must
be used with care. Eczema of all the anal and genital
region is much benefited by the use of alkaline baths
(Formula 27), in the manner described in the chapter on
the treatment of eczema of the trunk, and general eczema
with subsequent use of carbolized ointment (Formula 73).

Eczema about the female genitals being often due to
discharges from the vagina or uterus some care must be

taken in the discovery and treatment of such causes, if they exist. In addition to the general and constitutional measures required, vaginal injections of various kinds may be necessary before eczema of the more external parts can entirely be removed. For this purpose my most common agent is carbolic acid, used in the strength of half a drachm to a drachm in a pint of water, this serving both to check leucorrhœal discharge and to act moderately as an antipruritic; chlorate of potassa or other measures suitable to the case may also be required, and when eczema in this region in females proves at all obstinate careful search should be made as to the condition of the deeper parts. The same principles of local treatment which have been already detailed, prevail here as well as in the cases previously described. Hot water is of the utmost value, and may be employed even to the extent of introducing the cloth a slight distance within the vulva. When ointment is applied it should be spread, as directed before, upon the woolly side of lint and the fold thrust very deeply between the labia and allowed to project externally, so as to reach to the full extent of the eruption. When there is very considerable deep itching without much external lesion, very great relief may be obtained from the ointment of chloral and camphor (Formula 71), used as freely as desired; this will irritate the parts if abraded, and cause a good deal of burning pain, but will very commonly arrest the itching. The liquor picis alkalinus (Formula 40) also will be found very valuable, diluted ten or twenty times, and laid between and on the affected surfaces by means of cloths wet with it. When there is thickening of the parts brisk frictions with caustic potassa, as previously described, followed by soothing ointment, give great relief.

The connection of eczema of this region with pruritus itself, depending upon glycosuria, must never be forgotten , and when there has been long-continued itching about the genital region, the urine should always be examined, both as regards sugar, and also to discover the other changes which are included under oxaluria, lithæmia, etc.

Eczema of the anus and genitals is not infrequently seen in children and often causes great distress before it is recognized. I have had cases which had been rebellious, but which yielded with promptness to the principles already detailed.

When considering the matter of diagnosis mention was made of the frequent occurrence of a vegetable parasitic eruption about the genital region, the eczema marginatum of former writers, tinea trichophytina cruris, or ring-worm of this region, and of the possibility of finding it associated with eczema. When this is discovered to exist we may at once use antiparasitic remedies, or it may be necessary first to treat the eczema element for a while, until the acute inflammation has in part subsided, in the manner previously detailed, and afterwards the parasiticide may be applied without causing irritation. The remedy which I most frequently resort to for the destruction of the parasite, is the strong, undiluted sulphurous acid, freely bathed on the part several times daily. When the diagnosis is correctly made, this will generally give immediate relief to the itching, and if persisted in, will singly and alone cure the case, although often other measures used in conjunction may, in some cases, accelerate matters. The acid may sometimes prove a little stimulating, and cause sharp pain for a moment if abrasions are present, but as a rule it is well borne, even by the most delicate skins. In order, however, to have good results from sulphurous acid it must be perfectly fresh, for if used as ordinarily found in the drug shops, it very likely has altered by constant exposure to the air, and the sulphurous acid, SO_2, has become sulphuric acid, SO_3, and is, of course, very irritating and not efficient as a parasiticide. For this reason I always have the patient

long standing and rebellious, it is advantageous
the part with an impermeable dressing, as oiled-
utta-percha, after the application of the sulphurous
ough there is danger if care be not exercised, of
; too much irritation thereby.

f the measures previously detailed may be used
ie to time, even when the parasitic eruption is
s adjuvants to the treatment. Not infrequently
ite will be found to have become deeply seated,
i removed from the surface the eruption may crop
i shortly after treatment has been discontinued;
:ason, it is always safe to continue the treatment
length of time, even after all active signs have
ideed, until even the staining has disappeared.

CHAPTER XIV.

THE MANAGEMENT OF ECZEMA OF THE TRUNK, AND GENERAL ECZEMA.

ALTHOUGH it is not very common to find eczema affecting the trunk alone, unaccompanied by eruption on other portions of the body, still this may happen, as no portion of the skin of the entire body is exempt from the liability of being affected by the eczematous process. It is not, however, at all infrequent to have an eczema of one part, say the head, hands, or feet, and at the same time one of greater or less extent upon some portion of the trunk. Here, as elsewhere, it may be either in the form of acute or chronic eczema.

Acute eczema is occasionally seen to follow the application of external irritants to the body, and not very infrequently results from the chafing of harsh or irritating underclothes, or from poisonous dyes in them. It will also at times develop quite acutely on the body, when other portions are affected, without any known cause. It may assume any or all of the phases of eczema, although vesiculation is not common, and, perhaps, the most usual form in which it appears is in the erythematous and papular, or erythemato-papular variety. We may have an acute and diffused eruption affecting a greater or less part of the body, the entire trunk being more or less thickly sprinkled with acute or sub-acute, raw papules of eczema. Or there may develop patches of any size or shape, of red, slightly thickened and roughened skin, often very raw, and more or less papular.

Upon the region beneath the mammæ, and about the

folds of the abdomen in fat persons we often have a moist eczema, exhibiting surfaces of a brilliant red color, and exuding a slightly sticky secretion, which, when seen may have partially dried upon them ; these surfaces are often very raw and very painful. In slighter forms this constitutes what is commonly called intertrigo, and is frequently seen where folds of the skin come in contact in fat infants and children, as more particularly described in the chapter on infantile eczema. In children and adults it may often be a purely local affair, from harsh usage or retention of irritating secretions, but is also not infrequently the lightest manifestation of the eczematous state.

In the axilla it is not at all uncommon to have a subacute erythematous eczema, exhibiting much the same features. But here we also occasionally meet with a form of eruption similar to that described in connection with eczema of the anus and genital regions, as eczema marginatum. This is not in reality an eczema, but is the tinea trichophytina or ring-worm of this region, which exhibits here the same features as dwelt upon in the connection alluded to ; these are the sharply defined and slightly prominent, advancing, red margin, with a tendency to clear in the centre. In simple eczema of this location we do not have the clearly defined margin, but the diseased surface merges insensibly into the surrounding skin, and is worse in the centre than at the periphery. Eczema of the axilla is often associated with or followed by abscesses which may be of greater or less size, and may be the source of much distress. Sometimes they are quite deep and involve the lymphatic glands, but generally they are superficial, and appear to be connected with the sweat glands, which are unusually large and abundant in this locality.

Eczema of the breasts is sometimes a very annoying affection in nursing females ; but it is also not infrequently seen in those who are not nursing, or even in single

women. Hardy has remarked that scabies should be suspected when an eczematous eruption is seen upon the breasts
of women who are not nursing. This, however, is placing
the matter in rather too strong a light, for while it may be
the case in a certain number of instances it is by no means
always the fact that the eruption is thus caused under these
circumstances. A little careful investigation of other elements, as dwelt upon in other chapters in reference to the
diagnosis of eczema from scabies, will suffice to distinguish
the two, even when there is an eruption upon the breasts.
The first appearance of eczema is generally about the nipples, which will itch and give rise to annoyance, and a little
serous discharge will be found which dries into a crust, which
re-forms as often as removed ; the eruption may spread from
this so as to cover all the areola, or, indeed, it may extend
to any degree and give very considerable annoyance. One
or both breasts may be attacked, alone or in conjunction
with eczema of other regions. Many instances of what
appears to be ordinary cracked nipples are undoubtedly
cases of eczema of this region, and the pain caused by
suckling an infant when this exists is sometimes very great.
The diagnosis is not usually difficult, care being taken to
exclude scabies.

  Within the past six or eight years considerable interest
has been developed in the subject of eczema of the nipple
and areola of the breast since the publication by Sir James
Paget, in the St. Bartholomew's Hospital Reports, for 1874,
of an article calling attention to a " disease of the mammary
areola preceding cancer of the mammary gland." The condition of the skin was described as resembling chronic eczema
in certain features, with an intensely red, raw surface, very
finely granular, giving rise to a copious, clear, yellowish, viscid
exudation ; the sensations were commonly tingling, itching,
and burning. " In some of the cases the eruption has presented the characters of an ordinary chronic eczema, with

minute vesications, succeeded by soft, moist, yellowish scabs or scales and a constant viscid exudation. In some it has been like psoriasis, dry, with a few white scales slowly desquamating ; and in both these forms, especially in the psoriasis, I " (Paget) " have seen the eruption spreading far beyond the areola in widening circles, or with scattered blotches of redness covering nearly the whole breast."

Paget's paper was based on fifteen cases, and since then a dozen or more additional cases have been brought forward, more or less corroborative, by Butlin, Morris, Thin, and others. The skin has also been examined microscopically in a number of instances, as also the tumors which have occurred in connection with or following the skin lesion. From these studies it seems tolerably well shown that the disease on the skin is not a true eczema, but that it is a degenerative condition, probably a slowly advancing cancerous change near the mouth of the lactiferous ducts, which at a very early stage leads to irritative effects on the superficial tissues of the nipples and surrounding skin, and eventually penetrates into the substance of the mammary gland.

The comparative rarity of the connection is shown by the statement of Mr. Morris, that of three hundred and five cases of cancer or supposed cancer treated by him in the cancer out-patient department of the Middlesex Hospital up to the end of 1878, there were only the two cases which he reported; also at St. Thomas's Hospital Mr. Arnott failed to find a single instance of any connection between eczema and cancer of the breast in two years. I have met with exactly the condition described in one exquisitely marked case, and in two other cases I have seen superficial erosions on the areola in connection with cancerous tumors of the breast. In the typical case mentioned there was around the nipple a circular patch of about two inches in diameter of a brilliant red, with a moist exuding surface

very suggestive of eczema ; the nipple, however, was almost
gone.   The eruption had been considered to be eczema by
several well-informed gentlemen, and had received faithful
and judicious treatment to this end for five months or more
without effect.   In the other cases, while the skin condition resembled much that described by Mr. Paget, it did
·not occur to me to liken the lesion on the skin to eczema,
and I regarded the cases as very superficial forms of epithelioma.   I have seen many cases of true eczema - on the
breast which had no cancerous connections.   Those who
have described the condition in England have thought that
the eruption on the areola, for which the name of " Paget's
disease " has been proposed, could not be specially differentiated from eczema ; the presence of a lump of any size in
the mamma, in connection with a lesion such as has been
described, should always excite suspicion; and an early
operation of complete removal, both of the affected skin
and the lump, is advised by all who have studied the subject.

There are very many eruptions which could be con-
·founded with eczema of the trunk, and to avoid repetition
reference must here be made to the chapter on general
diagnosis, where the differences exhibited between eczema
and other affections were dwelt upon.

Acute general eczema in the strictest sense of the word,
where the entire body is simultaneously affected, is a comparatively rare affection, although cases of it are occasionally met with.   Sometimes it begins very acutely with more
or less of febrile symptoms, and it may even be preceded
by a slight chill.   The surface becomes heated and itchy,
and shortly there is either a violent development of papules
or vesicles, or else large areas of acutely inflamed erythematous eczema appear.   It is not a very rare occurrence to
have a more or less general eruption of eczema develop
acutely in patients who have suffered from the disease in a

chronic form for some length of time. Exposure to cold, over-indulgence in eating or drinking, or great fatigue, together with some general local irritation, may combine to cause a large portion, or the entire surface of the skin to take on eczematous action. In these instances the eruption is more or less papular, usually the papules being quite scattered, and attended with a very considerable amount of burning and itching. When a very general eruption makes its appearance quite acutely, it commonly runs a tolerably short course, and may subside without leaving any appearance of chronic eczema. Very frequently, however, either separate patches remain or there may be a generally irritable state of the skin, with the occasional formation of papules which may last for some time.

Chronic general eczema is sometimes observed in very distressing forms. The entire surface of the body, from head to foot, is then the seat of a red, thickened, excessively itchy, and in many places raw eczema. Some of these cases have lasted for months or years before relief is obtained. When the eruption takes this form the differential diagnosis between it and dermatitis exfoliativa, or pityriasis rubra is difficult ; indeed, it is sometimes almost impossible to decide the question except after a careful and prolonged study of the case. Pityriasis rubra is characterized, however, by a dry condition of the skin from first to last, with the exfoliation of thin and papery patches of epidermis. There is not the amount of infiltration seen in eczema ; there is not the fissuring at the joints, nor is there the itching, burning, and pain which is attendant upon eczema. The more acute cases of general eczema sometimes very closely resemble other more common diseases, and here again reference must be made to the chapter on the general diagnosis of eczema.

Except when the result of direct irritating agents, eczema of the trunk, or general eczema is always of considerable import, as an indication of the condition of the general

health; it always shows a state of lowered vitality, and if
the warning is heeded and proper measures adopted, including perhaps rest and change of scene, the advent of the
disease may be a source of real gain to the patient. This
remark is true to a greater or less extent of all cases of
eczema which are at all severe; it is far better for the
patient that the skin should exhibit the signs of break
down than that these should be manifested first in one of
the internal organs more closely connected with the immediate life processes. Local agents appear to be operative to the least extent in most cases of eczema of the
trunk ; we do not have the constant irritation produced by
elements such as have been spoken of in connection with
eczema of the face and hands. Nor is there the factor of the
retarded circulation, as in eczema of the lower extremities;
nor yet do we recognize as a cause the loaded portal circulation, combined with local irritation or friction, which exists in connection with eczema of the anus and genital
regions. But when eczema occurs on the trunk it often
indicates profound disturbance of the functions of nutrition,
and when at all severe, is a lesion of some significance; its
internal treatment and management should therefore receive
the strictest attention.

The internal remedies to be employed in eczema of the
trunk do not differ greatly from those applicable to cases
where the eruption appears elsewhere; except as before
stated, that there is far more often a debility which will
require powerful tonics during the later period, or even at
the beginning of treatment. Moderate action of the
bowels should be secured by such means as have been
alluded to, while if there has been a state of habitual constipation the constant stimulation of the intestinal excretion by the aloes and iron pill (Formula 14) may be required for awhile. Generally such cooling mixtures as that
of magnesia or acetate of potassa (Formulæ 1, 2) are re-

quired, according to the case ; but very shortly the more powerful tonics with arsenic and iron (Formulæ 9, 10, 11) are demanded, often with the addition of strychnine and quinine; or, in connection with the first mentioned mixtures, the pill of iron and potassa (Formula 17) may be given, just before eating.

When the eczema of the trunk is at all severe, especially in case it is of the papular form, alkaline baths (Formula 27) are of the very greatest service. The patient may take these with advantage even as often as every night, or every other night, and later once or twice a week. The bath should be of a temperature neither too hot nor too cold, although it is preferable to have it a little warm than the reverse. The temperature may range from 88° Fahr. to 98°, according to the feelings of the patient and the season of the year. Ordinarily fifteen or twenty minutes duration will suffice ; but where there is much thickening or very great itching, the time may be prolonged to half an hour, a little hot water being added, if necessary, to prevent the patient from becoming chilled. The surface should be dried with as little friction as possible ; and for this purpose I have the body quickly enveloped in a sheet which has been thoroughly heated, and the drying accomplished by patting the sheet upon the part, rather than by any rubbing.

But it is often even more serviceable not to dry the surface at all until after the use of the application next to be described: This consists of the glycerite of starch, with carbolic acid (Formula 73), which latter may be varied in quantity according to the case; five grains to the ounce is usually sufficient to allay the itching, but ten or more may be required. The patient, rising in the bath while still wet, and standing in the water to prevent a chill, takes a considerable portion of the ointment upon the hands, and rubs them quickly together, and then lightly over the surface. A fresh portion is then taken and similarly applied elsewhere, and perhaps a third quantity, and the body is then gone over again with the hands, gently rubbing it into all portions of the surface, both that which is diseased and into the healthy skin. If the application is too sticky, the hands may be dipped into the bath water, and the surface moistened therewith. After this operation there is little necessity of other drying, but the parts may be further dried with the heated sheets, as before mentioned, if required, but much friction, as with a towel, should be avoided.

It is generally advisable to make some such application after the use of alkaline baths in all cases, inasmuch as the alkali not infrequently leaves the skin a trifle too dry and harsh, so that sometimes harm rather than good may result. Where the eruption is not very extensive, the parts can be dried before this application, and we may use much the same plan, substituting cosmoline or vaseline, carbolated in like manner, in place of the glycerite of starch. It is not necessary to apply a great amount of this, as the surface is to be simply smeared gently over with it, and it is to be rather well rubbed in, but without severe friction. This application should be made in a thoroughly warm room, or the exposure may result in internal difficulties.

Alkaline baths, given in the above manner, are frequently of service even where the eczema is quite localized, as upon the face or one of the extremities. The action of such baths is not wholly confined to the diseased skin, but undoubtedly certain results take place therefrom which affect the entire processes of life. Aside from the direct absorption of the materials in the bath, there is an effect produced upon the system by the agency of bathing which is as yet unexplained; although the results have been observed and recorded, in the direction of hastened tissue metamorphosis exhibited in various ways, and most strikingly in the altered condition of the urine.

The local treatment of eczema of the trunk, or of portions of it, is sometimes quite troublesome to manage, because of the difficulty experienced in keeping the remedies employed in accurate approximation to the affected part. Some care and patience, as well as ingenuity, therefore, will often be required to adjust and maintain sufficient and proper support and protection for affected portions of the trunk, and the physician must see to it that this is accomplished, for if left entirely to the patient it will often be found that the desired end has been quite frustrated by the method of carrying out the plan proposed.

Eczema beneath the breasts, although very severe, will sometimes yield very quickly indeed to a complete separation of the parts by means of a fold of linen or lint spread thickly with a weak zinc or bismuth ointment; the cloth being twice the size of the eruption, it is to be doubled over and laid between the parts, so that ointment touches both sides. Powders are of little service here, as they work into a paste with the secretions, and thus may prove very irritating Later in its stage, eczema beneath the breasts may require some stimulation, and the compound tincture of green soap (Formula 41) is to be briskly rubbed over the affected parts, and the surface dried and the proper ointment reapplied; this will generally be all-sufficient. Care must be taken not to adopt this stimulating plan too early, or only irritation may result.

Eczema upon the nipples and breasts during lactation is often a very distressing affair, and the treatment is much interfered with by the nursing. It is, however, often quite possible to remove this, even while the infant still feeds at the breast. For this purpose, directly after the child has suckled, the nipple is gently dried by pressing on a soft, old handkerchief for a moment, and then the compound tincture of benzoin is painted freely upon the parts, and is allowed to remain and dry on; after this the surface may be covered with a little weak zinc or bismuth ointment.

This will frequently be sufficient, but if there are fissures which are rebellious, they should be touched with a pointed stick of nitrate of silver, and the nitrate of lead, in ointment, half a drachm to the ounce, forms a good subsequent dressing ; or the surface may be treated as before described, and any of the previously mentioned modes of treatment may be required in certain cases. Much may be done to prevent the occurrence of the cracked nipples and consequent eczema by the most careful cleanliness, and the application of the mother's saliva after nursing ; also by the occasional use of brandy saturated with borax, applied several times daily.

Eczema in the axilla, which may give the patient great annoyance, will often yield very quickly to a thorough and continuous application of the tannin ointment, half a drachm or a drachm to the ounce, or a mild zinc or bismuth ointment, and the avoidance of washing. The itching is sometimes very severe in this location, and the tar and zinc ointment (Formula 57) will often prove of great service. Where furuncles or abscesses appear with the eczema, they are to be treated in the ordinary way, with poultices if painful and if inclined to suppurate, though frequently they will disappear without opening under the continuous use of one of the ointments mentioned. The internal use of the sulphide of calcium, or the hyposulphite of soda, must never be forgotten when there is a furuncular tendency in eczema. As before mentioned, the parasitic disease, eczema marginatum, or ring-worm, may be developed in the axilla, and should be recognized and treated in the same manner as described in the chapter on eczema of the anus and genital region. When it exists unrecognized, the eruption may last for a long time, and prove rebellious to an otherwise well-directed treatment.

General eczema requires careful handling ; when it develops acutely there is commonly more or less fever and considerable prostration, and almost all local measures will seem to irritate. In the most acute stages powders are of the greatest value; the entire surface may be enveloped or very freely dusted with buckwheat flour, powdered starch, or ordinary flour, alone or combined with astringents (Formulæ 23, 24, 26). If there is much burning and itching camphor may be added to the powder, or, chloral may also be combined with camphor and used with powdered starch with excellent effect (Formula 25). This, however, does not yield a powder which can be dusted on, but it is a little heavy and sticky and is to be lightly rubbed over the surface. Very commonly, however, one of the simple powders referred to, as buckwheat flour, will be found to be more agreeable and cooling than those combined with medicaments; that is, if proper internal measures have been attended to.

When there is much exudation a powder does not answer very well as it is liable to crust up with the exudate and cause the clothing and bedding to adhere to the diseased surface, causing great distress. Here we have a valuable remedy in the external application of oil, and for this purpose cod-liver oil or linseed oil is the best; vaseline or cosmoline may be also thus used, but I have not been as pleased with their action as with the last mentioned. The entire body may be brushed lightly over with the oil as many times as is necessary, and cloths soaked with it may be laid upon the part; the linimentum calcis (Formula 48) is also at times serviceable for the same purpose. In somewhat later stages, when there is scaling and more itching, the addition of oil of cade to the oil employed (Formula 49) is of the greatest value; sometimes this may be a little too stimulating, but the proportions may be varied to suit the feelings of the patient. The addition of a small amount of carbolic acid, five or ten grains to the ounce or more, aids in allaying the itching. The diachylon ointment, if perfectly and freshly made, forms a good application in general eczema, and I have seen patients kept enveloped in it for considerable periods, in Vienna. But ointments are difficult of application when large surfaces are affected, and the great quantity required is an objection to their use; as ordinarily given for patients to apply at their own discretion they are very often very inefficiently used.

If the eruption is not too acute, baths such as previously described are called for. It is a mistake to wash the general surface when affected with eczema, with soap, as is often done. Even baths with the green soap, so commonly used in the treatment of skin diseases, will sometimes prolong a case which will rapidly yield to protective treatment. While small patches may do well under stimulation large eczematous surfaces are apt to be easily irritated. I much prefer to use the alkaline bath as described, well protected with starch. In the more acute stages, it may be best to increase the proportion of the starch very largely, and subsequent to the bath the carbolized glycerite of starch, or one of the petroleum preparations, should always be used. It is often very serviceable to save out a portion of the bath water, when prepared for use, to be employed for cleansing the parts at another time, if required.

In acute general eczema the diet should be light and unstimulating for a short time, and the bowels and kidneys well attended to. But in cases which have lasted any length of time the condition will be found to be one of very considerable debility; and in addition to care of the emunctories, we will often have to give powerful general stimulants. Arsenic is of very considerable value in the more general chronic cases, but it should be combined with other remedies, and is seldom of value alone. Cod-liver oil, internally, is also very generally useful. In eczema which is at all general, ale or beer, or much spirits should be most strenuously avoided. A small amount of distilled liquor may be allowed with meals, if required, but as a rule all drinks containing alcohol are to be interdicted.

CHAPTER XV.

THAT articles of diet have a direct effect upon the skin for good or evil I think there can be no doubt in the minds of those who have given any thought to the subject; and that hygiene, in the broadest sense of the word, can exercise a like effect is also evident. But these subjects have, as yet, received very little serious thought or attention from the profession, and very few explicit directions are to be found in the books bearing upon the subject of skin diseases. The matter following, therefore, represents to a very large degree the personal views and experience of the writer; and, although the subject is yet in an undeveloped state, enough is already known to admit of certain definite rules being given, which shall be of more or less practical value.

We will speak first of diet, and afterwards develop the subject of hygiene.

All are more or less familiar with the acute erythema or urticaria resulting in some persons from the ingestion of some forms of fish, particularly shell-fish; also, occasionally from strawberries, bananas, etc. Some individuals are so constituted that, whenever these are partaken of, the eruption will appear, while many others are thus affected only when the articles are stale, or when they themselves are in a peculiarly susceptible condition. It is also well known that in some persons crops of acne follow the free use of certain articles, as buckwheat, while those arising from gross indiscretion in diet, as from the partaking largely of fruitcake, mince-pies, sausages, cheese, nuts, etc., are of daily observation on all sides. We also recall the eruptions produced by the internal administration of some articles used as drugs, such as copaiba, quinine, belladonna, iodide and bromide of potassium, etc. The skin lesions occasioned by all these are transitory affairs, very evidently depending upon the causes mentioned, and disappearing, as a rule, spontaneously when the causes cease to act.

Now, just as these acute disorders of the skin are produced by acutely acting dietary causes, so a chronic error in diet can and often does induce, or at least keep up, a more chronic cutaneous lesion, which of necessity will return as often as a conjunction of causes acts with sufficient force. The most evident and well-recognized association of dietary error and chronic lesion of the skin is in the case of scorbutus, where the hæmorrhagic tendency in the skin and other organs is plainly due to the deficiency in the vegetable portion of the diet. A but little recognized, although important alimentary cause of skin lesions is the use of alcohol, which has been shown to be a most important factor in the appearance of the cutaneous manifestations of syphilis, as well as of other diseases of the skin. The free use of tobacco may also act very prejudicially in eczema, as mentioned in another chapter.

Exactly in what manner diet has its influence upon the state of the skin cannot, of course, be accurately stated at present; but from what is known of the acute skin symptoms previously alluded to, we may conclude that there are four methods by means of which this result may be obtained: First, we may have a direct irritating action from ingesta upon the stomach and intestines, giving rise to reflex cutaneous eruptions, resulting in erythema and urticaria, as in the eruptions from shell-fish, strawberries, and other articles alluded to. These eruptions sometimes vanish very promptly when the offending mass is rejected from the stomach, or removed by purgation. Second, we may believe that certain elements act directly upon the skin tissues, as probably alcohol, buckwheat, bromide and iodide of potassium, etc. Third, articles of diet may produce indigestion, giving rise to the products of imperfectly elaborated material, which then have a direct irritating effect by their circulation through the capillaries, as in the acne following indulgence at the table in such articles as pastry, cheese, sweets, etc. And, fourth, the error in diet may consist in the absence of certain elements of food, as in the case of scorbutus. This latter is most strongly illustrated in strumous eczema, in which a full supply of fatty matter will often alone restore the healthy condition.

Dieting, as ordinarily understood, represents a starvation process, which is to be continued, for a longer or shorter period of time, with a view, as it were, of starving out a disease. The definition of the word verb to diet in Webster's Dictionary is, "to eat and drink sparingly, or by prescribed rules." In the present connection, it will be readily seen that the word diet has a broader meaning, and signifies *such a regulation of the quantity and quality of the food and drink taken, its mode of preparation, and the time and method of its consumption as shall conduce to the restoration and maintenance of health.*

There is no question whatever in my mind that proper dieting, as understood in the above definition, is of the very greatest importance in the management of eczema. Not only are articles, which experience has proved to be injurious, to be avoided, but other articles, which are often erroneously avoided, are to be taken, in order to form a total of healthy life. Defective assimilation and disassimilation are beyond doubt important factors in the production and continuance of eczema, as has been abundantly shown in previous chapters. These defects are to be remedied, not by medicine alone, but by the regulation of every element which enters into the nutrition of the body.   Given perfect nutrition, and eczema disappears.   Perfect nutrition cannot be attained, then, by drugs alone, if the supply from whence the tissues are formed is in itself faulty.

Undoubtedly a healthy appetite and good judgment are reliable guides in the majority of instances for the maintenance of health ; but unfortunately every one does not possess one or both of these, and the surroundings of modern society will often greatly influence individual caprice in one way or another.   The patient with eczema has, in the vast majority of instances, committed errors of diet, and is still committing such, which, if they do not render the disease incurable, certainly retard its cure.   There is no doubt that the gouty patient has produced or aggravated his disease by the pleasures of the table, or by his mode of life.   There is no doubt that many strumous and rachitic persons have become so by their diet and course of living.   There is no doubt, again, that the neurotic patient has induced his condition to a very large degree by his habits and surroundings. Eczema is related to these three states, and in the strictest investigation of the diet, hygiene, and conditions of life, and in the proper regulation of the same will be found the surest road to perfect and complete restoration to health.

The first point alluded to in our definition of diet was a regulation of the *quantity* of the food and drink taken.   I am convinced that in no small share of the cases of eczema in private life, the quantity of food taken is rather in excess than in deficiency.   In answer to the question, often put, if these patients have dyspepsia, they will say that they are not troubled unless they eat too much ; and it will often be found that in these cases it is not the nourishing and healthful articles of food which are in excess, but such as are found in desserts. Witness the very common remark when a very tempting dessert is offered : " I have had enough to eat, but that looks very good ; I will try a little."   And so it is that the digestive organs are continually taxed just a little beyond their powers. Not every one discriminates between taste and appetite ; the taste is gratified long after the appetite is satisfied.

When the infant is overfed, through the indulgence of its mother whenever it cries, it rejects its food by a natural process, and thereby saves much sickness. The gourmand in China is said to take an emetic, that he may again enjoy the pleasures of the table ; but the refinement of to-day rejects this coarse method of getting rid of the burden, and relies on the dinner-pill, or the laxative mineral waters, to carry off food which should never have entered the stomach. The result of this over-indulgence is, that the digestive organs can do their duty but in part, and partly-digested food is hurried along and the products of imperfect assimilation are absorbed into the blood. The organs of excretion cannot eliminate the waste matter presented to them, and as a result we have sick headache, biliousness, and skin diseases, mainly eczema. Medicine is resorted to, which whips the organs into action ; the surplus is removed ; some relief follows ; the organs rest from the medicinal stimulation ; the over-feeding is continued ; the system is again burdened with new matter, and again the same process is resorted to. The result must be apparent to all.

It will be understood, of course, that I do not claim this to be the fact in every case of eczema, for many will be found where comparatively little—indeed, far too little— food is taken and assimilated. But it is often these very patients who will give the history of having previously over-indulged the appetite, and who have thus laid the foundation of an indigestion which then prevents further indulgence. There are also instances, not uncommon, where this has not happened, but where other excesses have been at work. Eczema is a disease owning many causes, all of which may lead to the same road of debility. We will begin first with the diet in infantile eczema, where we often see very striking errors committed.

In infants at the breast, too frequent feeding is, I believe, a common source of harm in eczema, if, indeed, it is not often the actual cause of the disease in many instances. Especially is it common for the mother to give the child the breast every time it cries or is restless with itching, which generally aggravates the already existing digestive disorder. The time of feeding should be regulated, and the breast given not oftener than every two hours.

But, again, the times of feeding may be correct, and the error may be in the quality of the milk, from the faulty diet or condition of the mother. In my inquiries I have generally found that mothers with eczematous children at the breast are in the habit of taking daily a larger or smaller amount of ale, beer, porter, and sometimes wine; or else large amounts of tea, generally for the purpose of increasing the flow of breast-milk. I do not allow these to be taken by mothers nursing eczematous children under my care, but substitute milk or oatmeal, or thin gruel for this purpose; milk is really the best food upon which the mother may form milk, and seldom do I fail to have it used freely. If not well borne at first, the habit of taking it can be acquired; frequently it will be necessary to add a little alkali, and I commonly employ the liquor potassæ, ten or fifteen drops to a tumblerful of milk. Very much more can be accomplished in these cases by carefully investigating the state of the health and condition of life of the mother, and treating her properly, than by medication given directly to the infant at the breast. I am convinced that dyspepsia and constipation in the mother are very fertile causes of eczema in the child, and should always be looked for and remedied. Not at all infrequently rich chocolate, taken to make milk, will disagree with the mother, and, by means of her indigestion, influence badly the eczema in the child; these errors in assimilation will often be shown by the presence of oxalates or urates in the mother's urine. Now, if these elements exist, if the mother's secretions, as from the bowels, kidneys, skin and liver, are not healthy, certainly the secretion of milk is not healthy, and thus can provoke a disorder in the child.

The subject of the occasional disagreement of the mother's milk with the infant is one which is so fully recognized that it might seem unnecessary to dwell upon it here; but however much it is appreciated and acted upon in relation to other diseases, it appears to be seldom thought of in connection with eczema, although in reality it is of the utmost vital importance. Prolonged lactation is sometimes a cause of, or at least an impediment to the cure of eczema in the nursing child; not infrequently, therefore, it will be necessary to wean the child and place it upon proper nourishment before the eruption can be cured.

In the case of nursing infants with eczema, therefore, attention is always to be turned first to the mother, and in a large percentage if not in all cases, errors of assimilation and disintegration may be discovered in her, or a debility, which must first be corrected before great and permanent benefit to the eczema in the child can be hoped for or expected. It must be remembered, however, that these errors are not always apparent upon a casual observation of the case, but often need to be sought for in the mother, as has been insisted on in another chapter where these states were spoken of as connected directly with eczema in the subject. In not a few instances the milk furnished by the mother is absolutely too weak to sustain the child properly, and other nourishment must be provided, or the milk improved through the improvement in the mother's health, or both. I therefore have very frequent occasion to prescribe for the mother, attending to her diet, exercise, hygiene, etc.; giving tonics or alkalies, or other suitable treatment; and the mother may take cod-liver oil with much benefit to herself and to the child as well.

When the nutriment from the mother is still too weak, cod-liver oil may be given, even to very small children with eczema, with most excellent results; or, where it can be obtained, cream in small quantities should be added to the nourishment of infants with eczema whose nurse-mothers are in poor health and furnish milk insufficiently rich. Or again, oil may be administered by inunction, either cod-liver oil, linseed, sweet, or almond oil being used. The inunctions may be practiced night and morning, a considerable portion of the surface being lightly coated with the oil, and gently rubbed until most of it has been absorbed.

Many infants with eczema are found to be fed very erroneously, either in conjunction with nursing, or in lieu thereof, and a change in diet often assists the management of the case wonderfully. Milk I believe to be the proper nutriment for a child under one year of age, and yet very few of those whom I see, use this food sufficiently and rightly. It may be necessary to add an alkali to obtain its perfect assimilation; a few drops of liquor potassæ, or a few grains of bi-carbonate of soda, or a teaspoonful of the milk of magnesia may be added to each pint. When the patient exhibits a strumous condition lime-water is best. Most of these little patients are, however, found to be taking too large quantities of starchy food, such as farina, corn starch, etc., and in many instances far too much sugar is allowed with the food. Sometimes in the desire to avoid starchy substances, animal matter will be given in much too large proportion; and I have seen very young children stuffed with beef tea, beef juice, or extract of beef to an alarming extent. Eggs are sometimes given too freely; often they seem to do harm if taken entire, but I have had very great assistance from the use of the yolk of eggs, one or two being given daily, either raw with milk, or lightly cooked.

No absolutely definite rules can be given with regard to the diet, as it must be more or less determined by the necessities of each case, guided by enlightened judgment. In the more acute forms of eczema the diet should be light and unstimulating, and the organs of digestion assisted, as mentioned elsewhere ; in more chronic forms a tolerably full and nourishing diet is called for, provided that the organs of digestion are sedulously guarded, that they be not choked.

When the child with eczema has passed beyond the period of nourishment at the breast, great care is required that its diet be correct. I need hardly allude to the impropriety of giving young children "a little of all that is going," as I see daily done among the poor, and sometimes even among the educated classes. It must be remembered that the servants, to whom the care of children is often too largely committed, are generally taken from the lower walks of life, and are totally ignorant of all principles of health and life. Unless the matter of diet is regulated, it will frequently be found that even children at the breast are fed from the table with the food of adults, and especially do they often get a little tea or coffee, of which children are universally fond. These should of course be interdicted to all children, and they should be encouraged to use milk freely. Even among patients in the better ranks of society, I have found very young children also indulging in the most improper mode of living, not only in the way of large quantities of candy, chocolate, cake, etc., but even pickles, nuts, and most indigestible articles, with the utmost freedom. I am positive that the severest restrictions in these respects have been followed in my hands by results which had not been and could not be attained under previous treatment, which in itself was quite otherwise proper, until these causes of disease were removed; and yet I could give many instances where very intelligent persons were feeding patients with infantile eczema in a most outrageous and inexcusable manner, without the slightest check from their medical adviser.

It is almost a constant observation of mine that patients with eczema, of all ages, dislike or avoid fat as an article of diet; and from the results commonly obtained by means of cod-liver oil, I have long been convinced, and acted upon the idea, that absence of fat was an important etiological factor in eczema. I therefore insist that patients with this disease shall increase the use of fat as an article of food to the fullest extent possible with healthy digestion. But it must be clearly understood that this does not refer to fat in combination with other substances, as in articles fried, gravies, pastry, etc., but has reference to pure oily matter, as found in the fat of roast beef and mutton, also in butter, cream, etc. Some little care, however, must be exercised in executing this order to use fat largely by those not accustomed to it, because there is the danger of the production of a set or group of symptoms commonly known as bilious, as is very frequently seen in those who begin with cod-liver oil in too large doses. Alkalies are very commonly required to assist in its digestion; and it is also exceedingly important that the patient take as much open out-door exercise as possible, to produce complete combustion of the fat.

While fat is of value as an element of diet in eczema, other hydro-carbons, namely, starch and sugar, are to be diminished in the dietary; and this is especially to be attended to in cases exhibiting elements of a gouty state. Indeed, these patients will generally appreciate that over-indulgence in sweets and starches is very commonly followed by an aggravation of the eruption.

Another element of diet which often is required to be

supplied to eczema patients is a proper proportion of the truly nutritive portion of wheat, which is so commonly taken out and thrown away. In the ordinary process of preparing flour a considerable portion of the outer coating of the wheat is removed, and the patient thereby loses much of the phosphates, gluten, etc., so that the finer grades of flour consist of little more than pure wheat starch, and the ash resulting from burning them is almost pure carbon. To obtain the best results in eczema, not only must we diminish the quantity of the starch, but must increase the proportion of the elements which go to form the human frame. To accomplish this we need to employ the coarser grades of flour, or, what is yet better, a flour made by the new process, whereby only the silex coat is removed from the wheat kernel, which is then ground into flour. This forms a dark bread, highly nutritious, easily digestible, and acceptable to most patients. It need not be insisted upon as the sole bread they shall employ, but should be used to as great an extent as is compatible with reasonable comfort and pleasure.

It is well also to encourage largely the use of crushed wheat for breakfast, and, for a change, one may take without harm, hominy, rice, gluten, or corn meal; it is better, however, to use the cracked wheat as largely as possible. It is essential that it should be thoroughly cooked, and my common instruction is to have it boiled over-night and then again the second time in the morning. Oat meal is popularly regarded as " heating," and my impression is very strong that eczema patients do better without much or any of it, although I cannot well define exactly in what manner it acts disadvantageously.

It is often of service in cases of more acute eczema to limit the amount of meat taken. My observations have convinced me that in the main too much meat is consumed by a large share of those who can obtain it in this country.

When the urine is loaded with urates, an excess of nitrogenized food but augments this condition; and when the skin is in an inflamed and heated condition, with acutely developing eczema, a limitation of the meat taken to once, or at the most twice a day, is of great service. Indeed, not very infrequently it will be found of value to cut off the meat entirely, and to place even the adult patient upon a milk diet. It is an error to believe that the child suffering from eczema is benefited by the administration of a large amount of nitrogenous nourishment, or by stimulants. The processes of assimilation are commonly at fault, and an excess of highly nitrogenized food but clogs the over-burdened kidneys, whose function it is to eliminate a large share of those elements. A moderate amount of beef-juice (one or two teaspoonfuls), once daily, to an eczematous child of one or two years of age, is all that can be properly cared for; and in a majority of these cases cod-liver oil is far more serviceable.

It is supposed by many that fish is injurious and should be restricted in eczema. This is founded upon the fact previously alluded to, that in certain individuals some varieties of fish, especially shell-fish, call forth an eruption of erythema or urticaria. I have not found fish or shell-fish to be injurious in eczema, unless, indeed, there is a peculiar idiosyncrasy against them; although, of course, if the articles are stale, irritative effects may follow in eczema patients as well as in any others. I constantly order fish as an article of diet to take the place of meat, especially for eczematous subjects exhibiting nervous symptoms.

Fermented liquors, such as ale, beer, and wine, are undoubtedly harmful in eczema, and should be restricted, if not entirely avoided, in the vast majority of cases. I do not believe that it is the alcohol alone in the substances which does the harm; and, if necessity requires, it is far better to take a very small proportion of alcohol in the form of whiskey or brandy, properly diluted, with the meals, than the articles referred to. This, of course, applies specially to cases exhibiting the gouty habit, and particularly to those who have already experienced over-indulgence in this particular. A well-marked case of gouty eczema cannot possibly be cured thoroughly and permanently where the usual amount of these stimulants is resorted to. It must here be remembered that judgment is to be exercised in the matter of withdrawing stimulants from those who have been greatly accustomed to them, otherwise more harm than good may result; though it is safe to say that in the greater majority of instances they can be very largely, if not entirely, abandoned without deleterious results, their place being often fully supplied by proper tonics. The following list exhibits, perhaps, the relative harmfulness of this class of articles as it has appeared to me clinically : Ale, champagne, lager beer, cider, port wine, madeira wine, sherry, claret, white wines—they being named in the order of their harmfulness, beginning with the first. There does not appear to be so much difference between the distilled liquors, and it seems that it is rather the quantity than the quality which does the harm. If I ever allow these to be used in eczema, it is always strictly in accordance with the prescribed rule that they be taken by accurate measurement, to the extent of but a few teaspoonfuls once or twice daily, well diluted, with the meals.

Tea and coffee are commonly supposed to be injurious in eczema, and, to a certain extent, rightly so. Tea I find to be far more harmful than coffee, perhaps because it is more common for it to be taken in excess. I cannot speak with regard to the effect of large amounts of coffee. I am very confident that tea, if used in excess, is certainly harmful in eczema, and I continually find patients with this disease who are in the habit of consuming large amounts of this article; especially is this true among such persons as dressmakers, cooks, and others, who are much in-doors. In moderation neither tea nor coffee appears to have a decided influence upon eczema; and it is my custom to allow a single cup of coffee and one of tea, each once a day, but neither twice. I especially object to after-dinner coffee for eczema patients.

I have had good reason to believe that soup, as ordinarily taken, is not good as an article of diet to eczema patients. It seems to act injuriously by a dilution of the gastric juice, and possibly the greasy constituents of soup as ordinarily used act as a cause of indigestion; certain it is that many patients state that they are more troubled with heat, burning, and itching in eczematous parts after considerable indulgence in soups.

There are some few articles in the vegetable line which must also be attended to, as having probably a harmful influence in eczema. These are sweet potatoes and cabbage; also bananas, and many apples. It is also better, as a rule, to avoid all that is commonly known as salt food, such as corned beef, ham, salted fish, etc., although this is not absolutely necessary, and a little salt fish or bacon may even be taken as a relish with impunity.

The proper diet, therefore, in obstinate cases of eczema, as before intimated, is one which is both wholesome and nutritious in the strictest sense of the word. The necessaries of life are to be used as freely as are required, but care must be exercised in regard to many of the so-called luxuries, because commonly we find in them the source of the greatest harm to eczema. Chiefly to be interdicted are such articles as those into whose substance fat is burned, as in articles richly fried, of which fried oysters, fried egg-plant, crullers, doughnuts, etc., stand as types of the worst. With these must be forbidden the use of pastry, rich cake, cheese, pickles, nuts, raisins, and very richly-prepared preserves, together with rich candy, and even such luxuries as soda-

water with the syrups. Hot breads are undoubtedly deleterious, and, as a rule, none should be taken by eczema
patients which is less than twenty-four hours old. A very
common direction of mine is that eczema patients shall
avoid both the beginning and the end of the meal such as
is common to many, and I even prescribe that they shall
dine off a single plate or course, avoiding soup, entrées,
and dessert entirely.

A second point alluded to, in our definition of proper
diet, had reference to the mode of preparation of food; and
this is a matter of some importance. That food should be
properly cooked is evident to all, and that this is not always
done is equally evident. It is an error to believe that meat
a great deal underdone is of peculiar value, and, from experience with the digestion of younger people and dyspeptics,
I am convinced that meat should be thoroughly cooked in
order to be readily and thoroughly digested and well assimilated. But the outer, burned portions are not desirable,
and as a rule should be avoided by eczema patients; as also
the skin of poultry and the stuffing, rich gravies, etc.
Mention has already been made of the preparation of
breadstuffs; care should be taken that these are not too
fresh, and that they are thoroughly cooked, not soggy, nor
sour. Attention has been called to the harmfulness of
fried articles, and this point should be investigated, inasmuch as very many are in the habit of having food fried in
place of being cooked by other means.

Many of the points here alluded to may seem exceedingly homely and, perhaps, out of place in a scientific
treatise; but it will be remembered that the subject under
consideration is the "management of eczema," and unless
all points which conduce to a perfect restoration of health
are attended to, our aim cannot be quickly and thoroughly
accomplished.

The next point in the definition given of diet refers to

the time and method of consumption of food and drink;
and this is a matter of vital importance. Irregular meals,
or those hurriedly taken, cannot conduce to health, and
stand as obstacles to a cure of eczema. Regularity should
be observed in the time of taking food, and the quantity
at each time should be as nearly as possible that commonly
consumed. A breakfast sufficient to give nourishment
and vitality for the day ; a light lunch to afford moderate
support during work ; and a comparatively hearty evening
meal, to make up for the wear and tear of the day, are requisite.
With children, of course, the hearty meal may be taken, and
probably is better taken, in the middle of the day, when the
evening repast should be relatively light, consisting of bread,
milk, etc., avoiding such articles as cake and preserves.

A point of no little importance, but one which is too
much ignored, both by the profession and the laity, is the
time occupied in the consumption of food. Rapid eating
is a source of very grave harm, and is a habit which is very
common in America. With rapid eating, of course, comes
imperfect mastication and insufficient insalivation of the
food. The process of digestion undoubtedly commences in
the mouth ; and an imperfect performance of the work
allotted to this portion of the digestive tract, must throw
undue labor on other portions and result in impeded
digestion. Many inadvertently take large quantities of
water or other liquid with their meals to hasten the process
of swallowing ; this should be especially avoided, and no
fluid taken while food is in the mouth. Very cold water is
especially bad, at or near meal time ; but any fluid with eating, beyond a very moderate amount, certainly dilutes the
gastric juice and impairs digestion. Hot water taken half
an hour before meals will relieve thirst and benefit any dyspepsia that may be present. Nor is it well to take the
tumblerful, as many do, just at the close of the meal ; the
result is the same, water or fluid taken soon afterwards must

and does act prejudicially. A common direction of mine is, that the patient diminish the quantity of fluid customarily taken at the meals by one-half; one cup of tea where two were taken; half a goblet of water where one was drunk. This may be again further diminished if the patient is still taking large amounts.

As a further thought in the same direction, comes that with reference to the teeth. A number of times it has appeared to me that imperfect grinding teeth, or their absence, have been an element of importance in the causation or obstinacy of an eczema.

Still another practical suggestion is, in reference to the mental and physical state before and after eating. Great fatigue, mental or physical, before meals, may result in imperfect digestion; the same, occurring after eating, has a similar result. In the case, therefore, of business men, and of those who are obliged to work mentally or physically to a great degree, it is far better not to take the hearty meal at noon, when this might act as a disturbing agent, but to eat more heartily when, at the close of the day's work, rest can be taken after eating. Mental strain and shock can undoubtedly arrest the digestion, as I have repeatedly witnessed. Close mental application too often repeated, immediately after a hearty meal, can cause indigestion. This, with the other practical matters which have been alluded to, must be taken into consideration, when the attempt is made to cure an eczema which has long resisted treatment.

HYGIENE.

If dietary elements are of importance with regard to the management of eczema, because they affect the state of the body, and, consequently, that of its diseased portions, hygiene, understood in its broadest sense, is also worthy of consideration for the same reason. It will be difficult, perhaps, to fully define all that can be understood under the term hygiene; but, in the present connection, it is used as referring to every element which can conduce to the general health and vigor of the individual.

First in importance must undoubtedly be placed exercise. Explicit instructions should be given to one affected with chronic eczema in regard to this, for the judgment of few patients will lead them to employ this agent properly or sufficiently. Simply to advise one to take plenty of exercise in the open air, will not suffice; for the judgment of the patient may differ from that of the physician as to what is implied by this direction. This subject must be seen to, and full directions given if any results are to be obtained therefrom. No spasmodic or irregular exercise will be sufficient; but steady, daily action of the whole frame can, and certainly does, conduce to the restoration of the health of eczema patients, and to the removal of their disease. Horseback exercise undoubtedly stands very high, but so few are able to take this, and it is so often limited by the season of the year, weather, etc., that it is not wise to rely upon it. Walking, however, is a mode of gaining exercise which the humblest and poorest patient can resort to; and if this is properly employed, it will result in sufficient good. But, here again it is necessary that the physician direct the amount of exercise and the hours when it shall be taken, which must, of course, vary in many persons according to their strength. This walking should not be an easy saunter, nor should the time occupied in shopping and calling be included in that taken for exercise. A brisk walk, graduated according to the health and strength of the patient, and slowly increased until a number of miles daily are reached, is what the disease requires. The preferable times for taking this walk are, of course, during the hours of day, especially when the sun is shining brightly, and in its rays. When this cannot be done, the time may be suited to the necessities of the case; for those who can take it, exercise between the hours of eleven and three is undoubtedly of the most value. All other modes of giving the body healthy reaction may, of course, be used, as taste and opportunity offers—rowing, gymnastics, etc.; but care should be taken that the exercise at any one time is not so much as will exhaust the patient and compel a cessation of the same for a day or more, as is frequently the case when long walks, severe horseback rides, boating, and other very active exercises are taken.

Massage can often be employed with great advantage to eczema patients, and a thorough rubbing and kneading of the skin and tissues will aid greatly in promoting the processes of life. Electricity may also come in to assist in cases exhibiting a nervous element, but its agency as a direct curative agent in eczema is not as great as might be anticipated from the frequent nervous relations of the disease.

Bathing ranks next in importance as a hygienic measure, and the eczema patient should see to it that the entire skin is in a healthy condition. I am convinced that too little attention has been paid to the skin as an excretory organ, and that if it is made to perform its part well, great aid will be given in the treatment of eczema. A large number of patients with eczema complain of feeling the cold, or of a chilly state of the skin with each change in the weather; and this is found to pass away under a proper treatment of the disease and of the skin as an organ. It will be understood, of course, that what is here said must be taken in connection with what has been stated in preceding chapters in regard to the injurious action of water upon eczematous surfaces. Harm could easily be done to a diseased part by the same measures which would give increased health to portions not afflicted with the disease. Caution must, therefore, be exercised against injuring diseased portions, while we are stimulating healthy parts. Alkaline baths, such as have been described in the chapter on eczema of the body and elsewhere, are, as a general rule, of more or less value; and the person affected, even with a localized eczema—as upon the head or hands—will receive benefit from the frequent use of such baths. These may be taken even as often as every night on retiring, although in general such baths need not be taken more than once or twice a week. As a further aid to the skin, it is well, after them, to anoint the whole body with glycerite of starch, either alone or combined with a little carbolic acid, five or ten grains to the ounce; or with vaseline or cosmoline, as previously detailed. The daily cold or tepid sponge bath on arising, with good earnest friction thereafter, is also oftentimes very valuable, if there is a perfect reaction afterwards; if, however, the hands and feet are cold, and the circulation is poor after its use—a state which is common enough in eczema patients—this measure does not do good. The effect of bathing in any manner is not confined wholly to the skin, but results in an increased interchange of tissue elements throughout the entire body, as has been demonstrated by physiological experiments. It is for this reason that they are advised in eczema, as well as for their local effect upon the diseased portion of the skin, or upon the entire skin as an organ.

The subject of the effect and value of mineral waters in the management of eczema is one of very great interest, and one which requires still much study and clinical research; the statements extant with reference to their action are all too indefinite, and too many of them are from those whose experience is limited to one spring, and who are therefore in a measure biased in judgment.

My observations have been both of a negative character as well as positive, for it has fallen to my lot to see scores or hundreds of cases who have visited mineral springs either with no benefit, or with but temporary gain, or who were even made much worse thereby; while I have also seen a certain number who have been very greatly benefited, and only a few who were apparently cured by the proper employment of this means, when judiciously directed. To be of real service, the mineral water should be as intelligently prescribed as any other remedy ; certain springs are of value in certain forms of the disease or conditions of the system, while in other cases a very different mineral water is required. Failure to discriminate in this matter, has led to innumerable disappointments and fruitless journeys at vast trouble and expense.

Another cause of failure in connection with the employment of these means of healing, which nature has scattered so lavishly in this and foreign lands, is too often the neglect of other and proper measures at the same time and in connection with the proper employment of the mineral water. This refers to diet, hygiene and other treatment, local and general, as indicated in this and other chapters. Not only should the life and condition of the patient be directed, together with the proper employment of the waters, as to hours of drinking and the quantity, also in regard to the hours, duration, and mode of bathing; but in many instances internal remedies can be employed to the very best advantage in conjunction with a treatment by mineral waters, while proper local treatment of the affected parts is essential to success in a large share of cases. On the other hand, much of the good obtained from visits to mineral springs, can be directly counteracted by wrong living there, or by erroneous treatment and irritation of the diseased portions.

In regard to the relative value of the mineral waters of this country and Europe, there is no doubt whatever but that equally good springs may be found here as abroad, possibly better ; but this branch of therapeutics has been far too little studied in this country, whereas the

springs of Europe have been resorted to for centuries
by thousands of patients, and consequently up to the
ent time the characters and virtues of the waters have
more developed abroad than here. However, with s
and careful observation, our springs will soon be thorou
understood, and the indications are that the variety f
here will soon be much greater than abroad ; we alr
know of some which excel those in foreign lands, and s
exist which are different from any known elsewhere.

Moreover, it is far more the custom at the Euroj
springs than it is at those in this country, to cor
the resident physicians who have given more or
attention to the subject, in regard to the applicat
of the waters and the mode of their employment, ar
this way much better results are obtained, than wher
waters are used unintelligently, as is so often the
by those visiting our springs ; moreover, the applia
for using the waters are much more complete, as a
abroad than with us. Finally when patients go tc
springs of Europe, they are themselves much r
careful and willing to abide by the rules and regulai
which may be laid down, than appears to be the
in our own land ; witness the very few, even of t
who go by medical advice to Saratoga or other wate:
places who give particular heed to matters pertainin,
health, as relates to diet, mode of life, etc.

There is still another reason why a visit to one ol
mineral springs abroad, more frequently proves to b
service than a stay at one in this country. This is f(
in the complete rest and change afforded by the o
voyage, with perhaps, certain beneficial effects fron
sea itself, together with the rest, change of scene,
climate, etc., found in a foreign land. And it is
questionable if a large share of the gain experienced (
trips to springs abroad, may not be rightly attribute

these agencies, quite as much perhaps, as to the special action of the waters.

But if rightly used in proper subjects, mineral waters are of themselves of very considerable value in many cases of eczema, whether employed at home or abroad, although in very few instances indeed are they capable alone of effecting a cure. As an adjuvant to careful and complete treatment they often render efficient service, and when it is reasonably convenient for one suffering from eczema to pass some time in the summer at a proper spring, it may prove a great gain, both from the direct use of the waters, and by keeping the patient from an injurious locality, or by enforcing a vacation.

There are not many mineral springs of which we have much positive evidence showing their direct curative value in eczema, although there are a considerable number which have more or less of a reputation in this direction. From what has been said in this and other chapters, it may be readily understood that no one spring or class of springs, will suit every case, but that many varieties may be of service in different cases. There can never, therefore, be any one spring or even class of springs, which will be curative of all patients with eczema, and experience constantly verifies the fact that while one individual with the eruption has derived the greatest benefit from a visit to a special watering place, others will visit it in vain. It remains therefore to suit the mineral spring to the case in hand, just as other remedial measures must be employed with knowledge and discretion.

The alkaline sulphur waters, represented by Richfield, Avon, and the Greenbrier White Sulphur Springs in this country, Harrogate in England, and Baréges and Aix la Chapelle on the continent, have long had a considerable reputation in the treatment of eczema; which is undoubtedly well founded. They are especially serviceable in gouty and plethoric cases, in those of full habit, and those who have indulged in the pleasures of the table. The waters are drank, to the extent of producing slight purgation, and also bathed in ; it is generally desirable to supplement the action of these waters by a subsequent visit to those having chalybeate properties.

The saline waters and alkaline purgative waters have also a very considerable reputation in eczema, and assist certain cases; but their effect is more transient, and they are suited for more acute cases, where there is functional derangement of the liver and a catarrhal condition of the stomach and intestines.   This class of waters is repre- sented largely by certain of those at Saratoga, in this coun- try, and Epsom in England, with Kissingen, Homburg, Püllna, Carlsbad, and Friedrichshall among the waters of Germany; these are all of more or less service when drank from bottles at home.

Certain of the chalybeate waters are also known to be of value in proper cases of eczema; such are the Rock- bridge Alum, Bath Alum, and Bedford Alum springs of Virginia, Oak-Orchard Acid Springs in New York, and Schwalbach, and Spa in Europe.

The thermal waters are often resorted to for the cure of eczema, but they are of comparatively little real ser- vice.   Such are the Hot Springs of Arkansas and Vir- ginia, also the Warm and Healing Springs of Virginia, and Schlangenbad and Plombières in Europe. The effect of these waters is almost entirely due to the heat they contain, and it is very questionable whether, aside from the benefit obtained from the surroundings, rest, change of scene, etc., there is any more gain derived from the bathing in them than could be gotten from an equal amount of warm bathing at home. I have seen many eczema patients who have tried them with only temporary, if any, benefit, and do not know of any one who was ever cured by their means.

The brine baths of Kreuznach are sometimes resorted to for eczema, but from what I have observed their action is rather detrimental than beneficial, unless it be in strumous cases.

Finally, there are certain mineral springs which are of more or less service in eczema which can hardly be classed among any of the waters mentioned. Such are the Old Sweet Spring, in Virginia, whose action seems to be a pure tonic ; the Allegany Spring of Virginia which is of service apparently by reaching the dyspeptic conditions; the Berkshire Soda Spring, in Massachusetts, which has very considerable local reputation, but the exact nature of whose water is not yet known ; Vichy, in France, and Ems in Germany, which act by their alkalinity; and the Bourboule Spring in France, which, I believe, contains more arsenic than any other known.

It will thus be seen that the number and variety of mineral waters which have at times been recommended for and found of service in eczema is almost as great as that of the remedies which have been employed for this disease, and the secret of success with one, as with the other, lies in the proper adaptation of the remedy to the case. It would be preposterous to imagine that each and every one of the springs mentioned would be of service in every individual case, so different are they in composition, in their mode of use, and in their climate, surroundings, etc. ; and yet it is useless to deny that each and every one of them is or has been of value to eczema patients, for experience proves the contrary.

It follows, therefore, that much study and clinical observation is yet required in this direction, and much judgment and discretion should be employed in recommending one or another spring for eczema.

The analysis of the water is not always to be de
upon as a means of judging the value of the
for there is undoubtedly much efficacy in the
combinations found, and often ingredients whicl
for the least in the analysis have the most powerfu
clinically.   But a knowledge of the constituents
water, together with clinical observation and recor
the basis upon which therapeutical judgment m
grounded.

While the writer has very many observations re
in this direction he feels that it would be prema
attempt with the present amount of clinical reco
hand to attempt to mark out the line to be followe
than has been already done in what has preceded.

If properly handled the. mineral springs often
to be of great service in the treatment of eczema
as other diseases, but when wrongly employed the
be productive of harm ; or, at the very least, a
attempt often gives rise to much unnecessary troub
expense.   To simply advise a patient with eczema t
some of the mineral springs, without further dire
is likely to be as useless, if not as harmful, as to
sick person, utterly ignorant of remedies, to a dru
without a prescription.

Turkish and Russian baths are very frequent
scribed in eczema, but their real value is far below
commonly supposed, and not infrequently they prove
ful.   When the eruption is at all acute or extensi
inflammation is aggravated by them, and when it is
and localized, they appear to have but little effect.
the older, humoral pathology of eczema, it was thoug
the *materies morbi* could be removed from the
through the skin ; but with modern enlightenme
inutility of this procedure is apparent, while clinica
ricnce has taught us that practically but little is

plished by this measure. As a means of promoting the activity of the skin they are occasionally of service, but it is questionable if the powerful stimulation of its glands to action is not often followed by a corresponding depression, so that any benefit derived from them is temporary. The danger of exciting fresh outbreaks of the eruption by means of Turkish and Russian baths must ever be kept in view.

Sulphur vapor baths are also used by many in the treatment of eczema, but their efficacy is very doubtful; the same objections hold in regard to their indiscriminate use as in regard to the hot air and vapor baths, in almost a greater degree. While sulphur vapor baths are of value in the parasitic affections, they can also cause an eruption on the skin, which may run into eczema in one so disposed; and they will very readily excite a sub-acute eczema into an inflammatory state. In certain cases of chronic, papular eruption they may sometimes be used with advantage, but in the main should be avoided in the ordinary treatment of eczema.

In regard to the effect of visits to the seashore and sea-bathing in eczema there is still necessity for much observation and clinical record. Sea-bathing appears generally to be injurious to parts affected with the eruption, certainly to those at all acutely inflamed; but sea-air and sea-bathing are often very beneficial to eczematous patients, especially to those who have lived at some distance from the ocean. As a rule, those dwelling on the sea-board receive most gain from an entire change to a mountainous region.

Proper rest and hours of sleep should never be neglected by the physician who seeks to·cure a chronic and obstinate case of eczema, for they not infrequently form an important element in the patient's health or ill health. I have constant occasion to correct this matter, both m the case of children and adults, and feel confident that gain has resulted therefrom to eczema patients. I have also had reason very frequently to direct patients in regard to taking proper rest from work. In the cure of obstinate cases, we must often prescribe rest from physical and mental employment, because nervous influences can play an important part in causing and prolonging eczema. The direction of the summer vacation is, therefore, a point which I continually take under my care.

Ventilation and sunlight are also items which are often neglected by many, and should, therefore, not escape the careful physician's attention who seeks to cure an obstinate case of eczema. Sunlight is quite as necessary to the health and life of the human being as it is to the plant or flower. All know that these will not flourish well on the north side of the house, or if deprived of the actual rays of the sun, however light their surroundings may be. Foul air may be a factor in the acquisition of eczema. I have seen a number of cases of eczema in which I believed that defective ventilation and plumbing had a not inconsiderable share as etiological factors. These acted, perhaps, not so much as direct causes as by lowering the vitality, and thus inviting the disease. Dampness of an apartment may also have a bearing on the case; also too great dryness, as by furnace heat without evaporating water, can dry the skin too much and thus open the way for eczema.

Finally, no item which can conduce to the physical welfare of the patient is beneath the notice of the medical man who would successfully treat eczema. Diet and hygiene represent a large share of the elements of human existence, and are often, or rather always, more potent for health or ill health than what are commonly known as medicines; and what is true of the general economy, is still vitally true in regard to one of the most important emunctories of the body—namely, the skin.

CHAPTER XVI.

THERAPEUTICS OF ECZEMA.

In the presentation of the following prescriptions, and in the references to them in the text, it is not intended that they shall represent fixed formulæ, from which there shall be no deviation in practice, but they are given to indicate in the main the mode in which the remedies spoken of are employed by the writer. Individual cases vary so greatly that a certain amount of latitude must always be taken, and no hard and fast rules can ever be given for the administration of any drug, or the employment of any local application. The prescriptions here recorded, therefore, only represent the average method of use of the remedies which are of service in eczema, and in many, if not in most instances, they must be altered to suit the case in hand. The combinations must be used with discretion and knowledge, and in the light of what has been stated in previous chapters in regard to the nature and causes of eczema. The doses indicated are mainly for adults.

MIXTURES.

1. *Mistura ferri et magnesii.*

℞. Magnesii sulphatis, ℨ vi— ℥ iss	23	32—46	65
Ferri sulphatis, ℨ i.	3	88	
Acidi sulphurici dil., ℨ ii	10		
Syrupi pruni virginianæ, ℥ i	40		
Aquæ, *ad* ℥ iv.......................	120		

M. S. Teaspoonful, in water, through a tube, after meals; (or the same with the addition of strychnia, or quinia, or both).

2. *Mistura potassii acetatis.*

℞. Potassii acetatis, ℥ iv— ℥ iss .... 15|55—46|65
    Tincturæ nucis vomicæ, ℨ ii............. 7|50
    Infusi quassiæ.......................
    (*vel* Tincturæ cinchonæ comp.) *ad* ℥ iv... 120|

M. S. Teaspoonful in water after meals.

3. *Mistura ammonii acetatis.*

℞. Potassii acetatis, ℨ i— ℨ iii............. 3|88—11 64
    Spiritus ætheris nitrosi, ℨ ii— ℨ iv .... 6|75—13.50
    Liquoris ammonii acetatis, *ad* ℥ iv....... 120|

M. S. Teaspoonful, well diluted, on an empty stomach—of especial service for children. A small portion of aconite may be added in febrile conditions.

4. *Mistura diuretica.*

℞. Potassii citratis, ℥ i— ℥ ii .... 31|10—62|20
    Tritici repentis, ℥ ii.................... 62|20
    Seminis lini, ℥ i .... 31|10

M. S. Place in a pint of hot water, and when cold take two to four tablespoonfuls every three or four hours.

5. *Mistura stillingiæ.*

℞. Potassii carbonatis, ℥ i................. 31 10
    Tincturæ nucis vomicæ, ℨ ii— ℨ iv........ 7|50—15|
    Extracti stillingiæ fluidi, *ad* ℥ iv......... 120|

M. S. Teaspoonful, in water, after meals.

6. *Mistura antacida.*

℞. Potassii acetatis, ℨ ss— ℨ ii............. 11|94— 7|77
    Misturæ cretæ, ℨ ii— ℥ i............... 7|50—30|
    Aquæ anisi, *ad* ℥ ii .... 60|

M. S. One to two teaspoonfuls after meals, or as required; of especial value for children.

7. *Mistura rhei et sodæ.*

℞. Pulveris rhei, ℨ i— ℨ ii.................. 3|88— 7|77
    Sodii bi-carbonatis, ℨ i— ℨ iii .... 3|88—11 64
    Aquæ menthæ piperitæ, ℥ iv........... 120|

M. S. Teaspoonful, in water, after meals.

8. *Mistura acidi nitrici.*

℞. Acidi nitrici fortioris, ℥ ss— ℥ iii......... | 1|90—11|25
Syrupi zingiberis, ℥ ss....... .... | 20|
Aquæ, *ad* ℥ iv..................... | 120|

M. S. Teaspoonful in water, through a tube, after meals.

9. *Mistura ferri et cinchonæ.*

℞. Ferri et ammonii citratis, ℥ i............ | 3|88
Liquoris potassii arsenitis, ℥ i—℥ ii...... | 3|75— 7|50
Liquoris potassæ, ℥ ii—℥ iv........... | 7|50—15
Tincturæ nucis vomicæ, ℥ ii............ | 7|50
Tincturæ cinchonæ compositæ, *ad* ℥ iv... | 120|

M. S. Teaspoonful, in water, after meals.

10. *Mistura ferro-arsenicalis.*

℞. Ferri et ammonii citratis, ℥ i................ | 3|88
Liquoris potassii arsenitis, ℥ iss.............. | 5|65
Liquoris potassæ, ℥ ii....................... | 7|50
Vini ferri (Malaga) dulcis, *ad* ℥ iv............ | 120|

M. S. Teaspoonful, after meals.

11. *Mistura arsenici chloridi.*

℞. Liquoris arsenici chloridi, ℥ i—℥ iv...... | 3|75— 7|50
Acidi muriatici diluti, ℥ iv............. | 15|
Tincturæ ferri chloridi, ℥ ii—℥ iv........ | 7|50—15
Aquæ, *ad* ℥ iv..................... | 120|

M. S. Teaspoonful in water, through a tube, during or after meals.

12. *Mistura ferri et phosphori.*

℞. Tincturæ ferri chloridi,.....................
Acidi phosphorici diluti,.....................
Syrupi limonis,.........................
Aquæ, *aa* ℥ i .... | 30|

M. S. One-half to one teaspoonful in water, through a tube, after meals.

PILLS.

13. *Pilulæ hydrargyri, colocynth., et ipecac.*

℞. Pilulæ hydrargyri,............................
Extracti colocynthidis comp., *aa* gr. x 64
Pulveris ipecacuanhæ, gr. ii.................. 13
M. et divide in pilulas no. iv.

S. Take two at night and two on the second night after; to be followed each morning by a Seidlitz powder or Kissingen water.

14. *Pilulæ ferri et aloes.*

℞. Ferri sulphatis exsiccat., Ʒ ss................. 1|94
Pulveris aloes purificatæ, Ɖi................. 1|29
Pulveris aromatici, Ʒ i....................... 3|88
Confectionis rosæ, Ɖi....................... 1|29
M. et divide in pilulas, no. xl.

S. Take one or more after each meal, and diminish the dose and its frequency as rapidly as possible.

15. *Pilulæ rhei, sodæ, et ipecac.*

℞. Pulveris rhei,..........................
Sodii bicarbonatis, *aa* Ʒ ss—Ʒ i......... 1|94— 3|88
Pulveris ipecacuanhæ, gr. x............. 64
M. et divide in pilulas, no. xxx.
S. Take one after meals.

16. *Pilulæ hydrargyri iodidi.*

℞. Hydrargyri iodidi viridi, gr. x—xx....... 64— 1|29
Extracti conii alcoholici, Ɖii .... 2|59
M. et divide in pilulas, no. xl.
S. Take one morning and night.

17. *Pilulæ ferri et potassii.*

℞. Ferri sulphatis exsiccat.,.....................
Potassii carbonatis,...........................
Potassii tartratis, *aa* Ʒ ii..................... 7|77
M. et divide in pilulas, no. xlviii—lx.

S. Take at first one after meals, and increase up to three or more after each meal.

18. *Pilulæ arsenici et ferri.*

℞. Liquoris potassii arsenitis, ʒ i—ʒ ii......   3|75   7,50
    Ferri sulphatis exsiccatæ, ʒ i...........   3|88
    Sodii bicarbonatis, ʒ i—ʒ ii............   3|88— 7|77
    Extracti gentianæ, ʒ ss—ʒ i...........   1|94— 3|88
M. et divide in pilulas, no. xxx.
    S. Take one after meals.

POWDERS.

19. *Pulvis hydrargyri chloridi.*

℞. Hydrargyri chloridi mitis, gr. v—gr. xv.. |32 |97
    Sodii bicarbonatis, gr. x—gr. xxx....... |64— 1|94
M. et divide in pulveres, no. vi.
    S. Take one every morning ; for children.

20. *Pulvis sulphuris et potassii.*

℞. Sulphuris precipitati,..........................
    Potassii bi-tartratis, *aa* ʒ i...................   31|10
    M. S. One to two teaspoonfuls, stirred in water, on retiring.

21. *Pulvis manganesii et pepsini.*

℞. Manganesii oxidi nigri,.......................
    Pepsini porci, *aa* ʒ ii.......................   7|77
M. et divide in pulveres, no. xxiv.
    S. Take one or more after meals.

22. *Pulvis bismuthi et sodii.*

℞. Bismuthi subnitratis, ʒ i—ʒ ii. ....   3|88— 7|77
    Sodii bicarbonatis, ʒ ii.................   7|77
    Pulveris zingiberis, Ɔ ii.................   2|59
M. et divide in pulveres, no. xii.
    S. Take one after meals.

In preparing dusting powders for external use the
greatest caution must be exercised that they are in the
finest possible state, and entirely free from gritty particles ; those which contain mineral ingredients should be
shaken or stirred before being applied, as otherwise a
separation of the constituents may interfere with their ben-

eficial action.   Care must be taken that pov
allowed to cake upon the skin, or to become
a paste, as in the flexures of joints and elsev

23. *Pulvis camphoræ et zinci.*

℞. Pulveris camphoræ, ℈ss—℈i............   1
Zinci oxidi, ℥iv........................   15
Pulveris amyli, ℥i.....................   31
M. S. Use externally as a dusting powder.

24. *Pulvis magnesii carbonatis.*

℞. Magnesii carbonatis levis,................. ....
Pulveris lycopodii, *aa* ℥ss.................
M. S. Use externally as a dusting powder.

25. *Pulvis antipruriticus.*

℞. Chloralis hydratis,.....................
Camphoræ, *aa* ℈i.....................   3
Rub together until liquid and incorporate with
Pulveris amyli, ℥i—℥ii..............   31
M. Keep tightly corked in a wide-mouthed bottle
S. Use externally ; rub well on the skin with th

26. *Pulvis aluminii et amyli.*

℞. Aluminii acetatis, ℈iv.....................
Pulveris amyli, ℥iss.......................
M. S. Use externally as a dusting powder.

BATHS.

The capacity of bath tubs varies so greatly
sirable to have a fixed, definite amount to be
medicated bath, and if a larger or smaller
water is desired, a relative quantity of the ingr
be taken.   The amount calculated for in th
formulæ is thirty gallons.   The temperature :
somewhat with the patient, the season, and th
sired.   For the full bath, to be taken for an
time, the temperature should not go below

.86° Fahr. at the lowest ; the highest should not, as a rule, exceed 100° Fahr. In ordinary cases from 88° Fahr. to 94° Fahr. suffices, but care must be taken that the temperature is not so low that any chilling takes place, nor so great that the system becomes heated thereby. To obtain much effect from the bath, the patient should remain in it from fifteen to twenty-five minutes, or even longer, additional hot water being employed in cold weather to prevent much lowering of temperature ; children should remain in for a shorter time. The degree of heat belonging to various baths has generally been accepted at about the following figures : a *tepid bath* ranges from 85° to 92° Fahr., a *warm bath*, from 92° to 98° Fahr., and a *hot bath* from 98° to 110°.

27. *Balneum potassii et sodii.*

℞. Potassii carbonatis, ℥ iv .... 124|41
Sodii carbonatis, ℥ iii........................... 93|30
Boracis pulveris, ℥ ii .... 62|20
M. S. Use one such powder for a thirty (30) gallon bath, with half a pound or more of starch.

28. *Balneum potassii et glycerinæ.*

℞. Potassii acetatis, ℥ vi.................. 186|61
Glycerinæ, Oi—Oii.................. 640|— 1280
M. S. Use in a thirty gallon bath.

29. *Balneum ammoniæ et glycerinæ.*

℞. Spiritûs ammoniæ aromatici,..................
Glycerinæ, *aa* ℥ viii.......................... 320|
M. S. Use in a thirty gallon bath.

30. *Balneum acidi carbolici.*

℞. Acidi carbolici, ℥ i—℥ iv .... 30| —120|
Gelatinæ, lb. i..................... 373|
Aquæ. Oii..................... 960|
M. S. Use in a thirty gallon bath.

LOTIONS.

The same care which is to be directed towards the avoidance of coarse and gritty particles in powders to be applied to the eczematous skin, is especially applicable to those contained in lotions. The ingredients should be very carefully pulverized; when the lotion containing a powder is applied, the resulting deposit on the skin should form an even, smooth, and non-irritating coating. It should always be remembered that glycerine is not well borne by every skin ; when it seems to irritate in these lotions, its place may be supplied by other demulcents.

31. *Lotio calaminæ et glycerinæ.*

℞. Pulveris calaminæ preparat., ℨi................   3|88
Zinci oxidi, ℈i— ℨii....................   3|88— 7|77
Glycerinæ, ℨi—℈iii...................   5| —15
Aquæ rosæ, *ad* ℥iv...................   120|
M. et ft. lotio.

32. *Lotio calaminæ et cretæ (Startin).*

℞. Pulveris calaminæ preparat., ℨi.........   3|88
Cretæ preparatæ, ℨi ℈ii..............   3|88— 7|77
Acidi hydrocyanici diluti, ℨss..........   1|90
Glycerinæ, ℈ii—℈iv...................   10| —20
Liquoris calcis, ℥iii...................   90|
Aquæ sambuci, *ad* ℥viii...............   240|
M. et ft. lotio.

33. *Lotio bismuthi et amygdalæ.*

℞. Bismuthi subnitratis, ℈iss..............   5|83
Acidi hydrocyanici diluti, ℨss—℈i......   1|90— 3|80
Emulsionis amygdalæ, *ad* ℥iv.........   120|
M. et ft. lotio.

34. *Lotio nigra.*

℞. Hydrargyri chloridi mitis, ℨi.................   3|88
Liquoris calcis, Oi ....   480|
M. et ft. lotio.

35. *Lotio zinci et plumbi.*

℞. Zinci oxidi, ℥ i—℥ ii...................... 3|88— 7|77
    Liquoris plumbi subacetatis dil., ℥ vi.... 22|50
    Glycerinæ, ℥ i—℥ iii .... 5| —15
    Infusi picis liquidæ, *ad* ℥ iv............ 120|

M. et ft. lotio.

36. *Pigmentum plumbi (Squire).*
(Glycerole of the sub-acetate of lead.)

℞. Plumbi acetatis, gr. cxx .... 7|77
    Plumbi oxidi, gr. lxxxiv...................... 5|44
    Glycerinæ, ℥ i............................ 40|

Digest the acetate of lead and the litharge in the glycerine (heated to 300° in an oil bath) for half an hour, constantly stirring. Then filter in a chamber heated to 300°. Use diluted.

37. *Lotio plumbi glyceriti.*

℞. Glyceriti plumbi subacetatis, ℥ ii—℥ ii... 5| —20
    (Squire's glycerole of the sub-acetate of lead.)
    Glycerinæ, ℥ ii........................ 10|
    Aquæ rosæ, *ad* ℥ iv.................. 120|

M. et ft. lotio.

38. *Lotio boracis et camphoræ.*

℞. Boracis pulveris, ℥ i..................... 3|88
    Tincturæ camphoræ, ℥ i—℥ ii.......... 3|75— 7|50
    Glycerinæ, ℥ i—℥ iii.................. 5| —15
    Aquæ aurantii florum, *ad* ℥ iv.......... 120|

M. et ft. lotio.

39. *Lotio plumbi et opii.*

℞. Liquoris plumbi subacetatis diluti ....
    Tincturæ opii *aa* ℥ i...................... 30|
    Aquæ, *ad* O i................................ 480|

M. et ft. lotio.

40. *Liquor picis alkalinus.*

℞. Picis liquidæ, ℥ ii......................... 62|20
    Potassæ causticæ, ℥ i...................... 31|10
    Aquæ, ℥ v .... 150|

M. Dissolve the potash in the water and add slowly to the tar, in a mortar, with friction.

S. To be used diluted.

41. *Tinctura saponis cum pice (Hebra).*
(Compound tincture of green soap.)

℞. Saponis viridis,...............................
Olei cadini,................................
Spiritus vini rectificati, *aa* ℨ i 30
M. filtra et adde,
Spiritus lavandulæ, ℨ ii,................... 7 50
M. et ft. lotio.

42. *Spiritus saponis kalinus (Hebra).*

℞. Saponis viridis, ℥ iv....................... 124 41
Spiritus vini rectificati, ℥ ii............... 54
M. filtra et adde,
Spiritus lavandulæ, ℨ i 3 75
M. et ft. lotio.

43. *Lotio glycerinæ et potassæ.*

℞. Glycerinæ, ℥ i............................. 40
Liquoris potassæ, ℥ ii 60
M. et ft. lotio.

44. *Lotio plumbi et ricini.*

℞. Plumbi acetatis, gr. viii.................... 51
Olei bergamii, ℨ ss 1 94
Olei ricini, ℨ iv.......................... 15 55
Spiritus vini rectificati, *ad* ℥ iv 108
M. et ft. lotio, for the scalp.

45. *Lotio quiniæ et zinci.*

℞. Quiniæ sulphatis, Ɔ i 1 29
Zinci sulphatis, gr. x 64
Tincturæ cantharadis, ℨ iii............... 11 64
Alcohol absoluti,.........................
Glycerinæ, *aa* ℨ iv........................ 15 55
Spiritus myrciæ, *ad* ℥ vi.................. 162
M. et ft. lotio, for the scalp.

46. *Lotio cantharidis et capsici.*

℞. Tincturæ cantharidis, ℨ ii—℥ iv......... 7 50—15
Tincturæ capsici, ℨ ii—℥ iv............. 7 50—15
Tincturæ nucis vomicæ, ℨ iv........... 15
Olei ricini, ℨ ii—ℨ iv.................. 10 —20
Aquæ cologniensis, *ad* ℥ iv 120
M. et ft. "hair lotion."

47. *Lotio ammoniæ et rosmarini.*

R. Aquæ ammoniæ fort,..........................
. Olei amygdalæ express, *aa* ℥ i................. 30
Spiritus rosmarini, ℥ iv..................... 108
Aquæ rosæ, ℥ ii............................. 60
M. ft. "hair lotion."

48. *Lotio calcis et olei lini.*

R. Liquoris calcis,...............................
Olei lini, *aa* ℥ iv............................ 120
M. et ft. lotio.

49. *Lotio olei cadini.*

R. Olei cadini, ℈ iv— ℥ i.................. 20 —40
Olei morrhuæ......................
(*vel* olei lini, *vel* olei amygd. express.), *ad*
℥ iv............................... 160
M. et ft. lotio.

50. *Lotio argenti nitratis.*

R. Argenti nitratis, gr. v—xxx............. 32— 1 94
Spiritus etheris nitrosi, ℥ i.............. 27
M. et ft. lotio.

OINTMENTS.

In the preparation of ointments, too much care cannot be exercised in having the substances to be incorporated in the finest possible state, for more harm than good is often done by having coarse particles in an ointment which is to be applied to an abraded surface. The physician should therefore take especial supervision over the preparation of ointments, and should frequently inspect those in use by the patient. It is well to grind down any mineral ingredient first in a mortar, and to add a little sweet almond oil, making it into a paste, which is then to be added to the excipient. The greatest care must also be exercised that the material is perfectly fresh, for the least rancidity in the ointment renders it irritating.

51. *Unguentum zinci oxidi.*

℞. Zinci oxidi, ʒ ss—ʒ i.................... 1|94— 3|88
    Unguenti aquæ rosæ, ℥ i............. 31|10
M. et ft. unguentum.

52. *Unguentum bismuthi sub-nitratis.*

℞. Bismuthi subnitratis, ʒ ss—ʒ ii......... 1|94— 7|77
    Unguenti aquæ laurocerasi, ℥ i.......... 31|10
M. et ft. unguentum.

53. *Unguentum acidi tannici.*

℞. Acidi tannici, ʒ i...................... 3'88
    Unguenti aquæ rosæ, ℥ i.................. 31 10
M. et ft. unguentum.

54. *Unguentum calaminæ compositum.*

℞. Pulveris calaminæ preparatæ, ʒ ss....... 1|94
    Zinci oxidi, ʒ ss—ʒ i.................. 1|94— 3|88
    Unguenti aquæ rosæ, ℥ i.............. 31|10
M. et ft. unguentum.

55. *Unguentum aluminii acetatis.*

℞. Alumini acetatis, ʒ ss—ʒ ii............. 1|94— 7|77
    Glyceriti amyli, ℥ i.................. 31,10
M. et ft. unguentum.

56. *Unguentum bismuthi (vel zinci) oleatis (Anderson).*

℞. Bismuthi oxidi, ʒ ii........................ 7|77
    Acidi oleici, ℥ ii........................ 62|20
    Unguenti petrolei, ℥ ii + ʒ ii.............. 70
    Ceræ albæ, ʒ vi. .... 23|32
    Olei rosæ, gtt. vi........................... 48

M. Rub up the bismuth oxide with the oleic acid, and let it stand for two hours; place in a water bath, add the vaseline and wax, and when dissolved stir until cold and add the oil of roses. Zinc oxide may be substituted for the bismuth.

57. *Unguentum picis et zinci.*

℞. Unguenti picis liquidæ, ʒ i—ʒ iii........ 3|88—11 64
    Zinci oxidi, ʒ ss—ʒ i.................... 1|94— 3 88
    Unguenti aquæ rosæ, *ad* ℥ i............ 31.10
M. et ft. unguentum.

58. *Unguentum cadini et zinci.*

℞. Olei cadini (*vel* rusci), ℨ ss—ℨ i.......... 2|50— 5
Zinci oxidi, ℨ ss—ℨ i.............. 1|94— 3|88
Unguenti aquæ rosæ, ℥ i.......... 31|10

M. et ft. unguentum.

59. *Unguentum cadini et hydrargyri.*

℞. Olei cadini, ℨ i.................... 5|
Unguenti hydrargyri oxidi rubri, ℨ i—ℨ ii __3|88— 7|77
Unguenti aquæ rosæ, *ad* ℥ i.......... 31|10

M. et ft. unguentum.

60. *Unguentum hydrargyri compositum.*

℞. Olei betulæ albæ, ℨ ss—ℨ i.......... 2 50— 5|
Unguenti hydrargyri nitratis, ℨ ss—ℨ i... 1 94— 3 88
Unguenti hydrargyri ammoniati, ℨ i—ℨ ii 3|88— 7,77
Unguenti petrolei, *ad* ℥ i 31 10

M. et ft. unguentum.

61. *Unguentum diachyli* (*Hebra*).
(Diachylon ointment.)

℞. Olei olivarum optimi, ℥ xv............ 600|
Plumbi oxidi, ℥ iii + ℨ vi............ 116 62
Olei lavandulæ, ℨ ii............ ... 10|

Add the oil to two pounds of water and heat it with constant stirring; the litharge is to be slowly sifted in while it is well stirred, fresh water being added as required. The ointment is to be stirred until cold, and the lavender then added. In winter a slightly larger quantity of oil is required, to make a soft ointment.

Several writers have recommended a diachylon ointment made by melting the emplastrum diachyli with olive, linseed, or other oils, or with vaseline, in proportions sufficient to make a soft ointment. These combinations answer the purpose fairly well, but are inferior to that perfectly prepared according to the above formula, because in them there is a portion of the oily substance uncombined with the lead, whereas according to Hebra's formula all the oil and lard are thoroughly combined and decomposed.

62. *Unguentum picis et hydrargyri.*

℞. Liquoris picis alkalini, ℨ i.............. 3|75
(See formula 40)
Unguenti hydrargyri ammoniati, ℨ ii—ℨ iv 7|77—15 55
Unguenti aquæ rosæ, *ad* ℥ i.... .... 31|10

M. et ft. unguentum.

63. *Unguentum hydrargyri et bismuthi.*

℞. Bismuthi sub-nitratis, Ʒi...............   3|88

    Unguenti hydrargyri ammoniati, Ʒi—Ʒiv   3|88—15|55

    Unguenti aquæ rosæ, *ad* ℥i......   31|10

M.   et ft. unguentum.

64. *Unguentum hydrargyri nitratis.*

℞. Unguenti hydrargyri nitratis, Ʒi—Ʒiii...   3|88—11|64

    Unguenti aquæ rosæ, *ad* ℥i............   31|10

    Olei geranii, gtt. v. .... |40

M.   et ft. unguentum.

65. *Unguentum hydrargyri et zinci.*

℞. Unguenti hydrargyri nitratis, Ʒi........   3|88

    Olei cadini, Ʒss—Ʒi.................   2|50 — 5

    Zinci oxidi, Ʒss... ....   1|94

    Unguenti aquæ rosæ, *ad* ℥i ....   31|10

    Olei limonis, gtt. ii.................... |15

M.   et ft. unguentum.

66. *Unguentum hydrargyri oxidi rubri.*

℞. Unguenti hydrargyri oxidi rubri, Ʒi— iii.   3|88—11|64

    Unguenti aquæ rosæ, *ad* ℥i............   31|10

M.   et ft. unguentum.

67. *Unguentum ferri subsulphatis.*

℞. Liquor ferri subsulphatis, Ʒi.................   3|75

    Unguenti aquæ rosæ......... ....

    Cetacei, *aa q.s. ad* ℥i 31 10

M.   et ft. unguentum.

68. *Unguentum hydrargyri cum plumbo (Startin).*

℞. Plumbi acetatis,............................

    Hydrargyri chloridi mitis, *aa* gr. x.... .... |64

    Zinci oxidi,................................

    Unguenti hydrargyri nitratis, *aa* gr. xx.........   1 29

    Adipis recentis,..............................

    Olei palmæ rectificati, *aa* ℥ss.....   20

M.   et ft. unguentum.

69. *Unguentum zinci compositum.*

℞. Balsami peruviani, ℨ i........................ 5|
Zinci oxidi, ℨ ss............................... 1|94
Unguenti aquæ rosæ, ℥ i.................... 31|10

M. et ft. unguentum.

70. *Unguentum plumbi et stramonii.*

℞. Liquoris plumbi subacetatis diluti, ℨ i.......... 3|75
Acidi tannici, ℈ i............................. 1|29
Unguenti stramonii, ℥ i..................... 31|10

M. et ft. unguentum.

71. *Unguentum antipruriticum.*

℞. Gummi camphoræ,.......................
Chloral hydratis, *aa* ℨ i—ℨ ii........... 3|88— 7|77
M. Rub together until a liquid results, then
add,
Unguenti aquæ rosæ, ℥ i.............. 31|10

M. et ft. unguentum.

72. *Unguentum picis et belladonnæ.*

℞. Unguenti picis liquidæ, ℨ vi.................. 23|32
Unguenti belladonnæ, ℨ iv.................... 15|55
Tincturæ aconiti, ℨ i......................... 3|75
Zinci oxidi, ℨ ii............................. 7|77
Unguenti aquæ rosæ, ℨ vi .... 23|32

M. et ft. unguentum.

73. *Unguentum acidi carbolici.*

℞. Acidi carbolici, ℈ i—℈ ii................ 1|60—10|
Glyceriti amyli (*vel* unguenti petrolei,) ℥ iv. 124|40

M. et ft. unguentum. Use after bath.

GENERAL REMARKS.

In the application of therapeutics to eczema, more is to
be accomplished by a careful study of the patient in every
aspect and the adaptation of remedies suitable to the conditions found, than by the employment of any special pre-

The same is true in reference to local appl
order to obtain success in their use they must
the existing condition of skin, and a clear idea r
of what it is desired to accomplish, otherwise
remedy may be employed where a soothing anc
action was called for, or a mild application m
inefficiently in place of a stimulant.

In the main, it is better to have a compara
list of remedies and to acquire skill in their us
to have a large pharmacopœia with which one
acquainted. The necessity is not for a new
eczema, but for a more perfect knowledge of
already recommended, which, when rightly usec
with all known measures, are quite sufficient f
of most cases; new remedies soon take their p
those of older date, if indeed they are not dis
experience continually verifies that which scien
edge demonstrates, that there is no specific for c
it may be added that, from the nature of the
never can be one found.

Attention to details is of the first importance
and the good effect of even the best remedi
frustrated by failure in some particular in the n
of the case, while the best local application will
its end, or even do harm, if wrongly employed.
sion, therefore, it is urged that patient study I
eczema cases and to the details of management
the preceding pages, as only thus can perfect
nent results be attained in dealing with a large
cases of this most troublesome affection.

INDEX.

A

Abscesses associated with eczema, 19, 152, 279,

Absorbent powders in eczema, 139.

Acetate of aluminium, 250.

Acetate of potassium in eczema, 125, 161, 162, 197, 267.

Acne, diagnosis from eczema, 48, 189, 191.

Aconite in eczema, 125, 162, 272.

Acute eczema, 35, 37, 39, 125

Ages of 2500 patients with eczema, 12.

Air, irritating effect of, in eczema, 24, 117, 187, 317.

Alcohol as a cause of eczema, 292.

Ale, influence on eczema, 302.

Aloes and iron in eczema, 131, 197, 265.

Alkalies in eczema, 125, 161, 197, 267.

Alkaline sulphur waters, 313.

    tar wash in eczema, 169, 249.

Analysis of names applied to eczema, 34–45.

    of 2500 cases of eczema, 10–21.

Anatomical changes in eczema, 28–33, 76.

Aniline dye eruption resembling eczema, 5, 39.

Antipruritics for eczema, 134, 272, 275, 289, 324, 333

Anus, frequency of eczema of the, 16, 252

Aperients in the treatment of eczema, 125, 130, 197, 265, 322

Application of ointments, mode of, 140, 167, 201, 271.

Arms, eczema of the, 218, 225.

Arnica causing eczema, 119.

    eruption resembling eczema, 5, 39.

Arsenic harmful in acute eczema, 126.

    in eczema, 123, 125, 132, 268, 290.

    in infantile eczema, 163.

    not a specific for eczema, 123.

Arthritic diathesis, 94.

Artificial eczema, 35, 38.

    eruptions resembling eczema, 5, 39, 71, 206.

Asthma associated with eczema, 19, 93, 192

Assimilation defective, in eczema, 97, 99, 198, 252, 295.

Atmospheric changes, effect upon eczema, 24, 117, 187, 317.

Auditory meatus, eczema of the, 195.

Auricle, eczema of the, 195.

Axilla, eczema of the, 279, 288.

B

Baker's itch, 36, 38, 206.

Bandages, rubber, in the treatment of eczema of the legs, 230–242.

Barber's itch, 36, 188.

Basis of local pathology of eczema, 71.

Bathing, injudicious, harm from, in eczema, 159, 309, 310.

Baths in eczema, 126, 169, 274, 285, 316, 324.

    Russian and Turkish, 316.

    sulphur. 317.

Beer, harmful in eczema, 302.

Belladonna, locally as an antipruritic, 272, 333

Bismuth ointment in eczema, 167, 330.

Black wash in eczema. 248.

Blepharitis often a form of eczema, 198.

Blisters in the treatment of eczema, 145, 222.

Blood, alteration of, in eczema, 98.

Boils in eczema, 18, 109.

Bowels, condition of, in eczema, 128–288.

Breasts, eczema of the, 279.

Bricklayer's itch, 38.

Bright's diseases, relation to eczema, 116.

Brine baths in eczema, 315.

Buckwheat flour, locally, in eczema, 139, 289.

Burning heat in eczema, 21.

C

Cade, oil of, in eczema, 172, 272.

Calamine lotion in eczema, 139, 274, 326.

Calcium, sulphide of, in boils and abscesses accompanying eczema, 153, 195.

Calomel in infantile eczema 164.

Camphor in eczema, 275, 289, 324, 333.

Capillary disturbance in eczema, 4, 24.

CPSIA information can be obtained
at www.ICGtesting.com
Printed in the USA
BVOW09s0721270617
487925BV00013B/303/P